Transgender Health - Advances and New Perspectives

Edited by Carlos Miguel Rios-González

Published in London, United Kingdom

Transgender Health - Advances and New Perspectives
http://dx.doi.org/10.5772/intechopen.98020
Edited by Carlos Miguel Rios-González

Contributors
Silvana de Souza Nascimento, Luz Gonçalves Brito, Phaedra Cress, Dalia Costa, Miguel Miranda, Kelly Davison, Christopher Salgado, Kerstin Yu, Tony Shao, Edward Gheiler, Stefan Kenel-Pierre, Camilla Taverna, Massimo Di Grazia, Carlos Miguel Rios-González

First published in London, United Kingdom, 2022 by IntechOpen
IntechOpen is the global imprint of INTECHOPEN LIMITED, registered in England and Wales, registration number: 11086078, 5 Princes Gate Court, London, SW7 2QJ, United Kingdom

British Library Cataloguing-in-Publication Data
A catalogue record for this book is available from the British Library

Additional hard and PDF copies can be obtained from orders@intechopen.com

Transgender Health - Advances and New Perspectives
Edited by Carlos Miguel Rios-González
p. cm.
Print ISBN 978-1-80355-297-2
Online ISBN 978-1-80355-298-9
eBook (PDF) ISBN 978-1-80355-299-6

Meet the editor

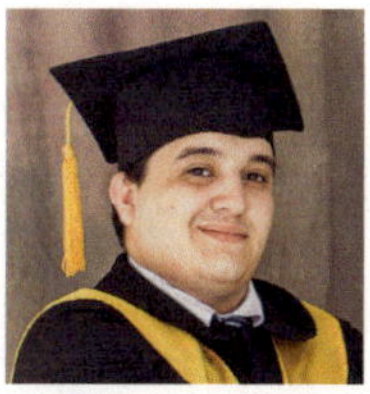

Carlos Miguel Rios-González is a medical surgeon with a specialization in health research, university didactics, infection control, and hospital epidemiology. He has a Master in Hospital Administration, a Master in Scientific Research Methodology, a Ph.D. in Public Health, and is currently pursuing a Master's in Higher Education in Medical Sciences and a Ph.D. in Education. Dr. Rios-González is the Research Director, Faculty of Medical Sciences, National University of Caaguazu, Paraguay. He is also a Researcher and Director of Education, at the National Institutes of Health, Ministry of Public Health and Social Welfare, director of the COCHRANE Paraguay Center, and president of the Health Ethics Committee – PY. He is an editor and reviewer of international scientific journals as well as an international speaker.

Contents

Preface

Sex and gender are closely related terms, however, they differ with respect to the corporality and identity of the individual. Sex responds to biological determinants of the individual (chromosomal or genotypic sex, anatomical or phenotypic sex), unlike gender, which responds to the internal personal experience of feeling masculine, feminine, or androgenous, depending on the cultural context in which these experiences are interpreted. Sexual orientation refers to who is the object of sexual-affective attraction (homosexual, heterosexual, bisexual, asexual, etc.).

Trans person is a general and inclusive term that encompasses those people whose gender identity and/or expression is different from the cultural expectations based on the sex assigned to them at birth. It includes transsexuals, transgender people, non-binary trans people, those with fluid gender expression, and other gender variations.

Trans people are made invisible and stigmatized and their reality is often unknown to society. They are often victims of violence and discrimination, which makes them especially vulnerable in the workplace, health, and social spheres.

The demand for health care for the transgender population is increasing throughout the world, both due to common health problems of the general population as well as the request for medical and surgical support in the process of transition towards sex felt by the person. Different health authorities have developed different orientations and care guidelines for this group of patients to safeguard care that respects the gender identity and expression of each person and allows for dignified treatment.

This book provides information on the social determinants and advances and new perspectives on health in trans populations. The first section is the Introduction. The second section addresses social determinants and includes four chapters. Chapter 2 discusses the experiences of survival and resilience of the trans population in Brazil. Chapter 3 presents data on related public policies in Portugal. Chapter 4 discusses the approach and accompaniment of transgender people, to start the transition process. Chapter 5 examines the health of trans people in Paraguay.

The second section focuses on advances and new perspectives and includes three chapters. Chapter 6 deals with the development of standards to improve the care of transgender people. Chapter 7 details the experience of phalloplasty in transgender men with and without urethral lengthening. Finally, Chapter 8 presents the effects of hypothalamic blockers in the treatment of gender dysphoria in preadolescence.

We extend special thanks to all the authors who contributed to this volume. We are also grateful to the staff at IntechOpen for their assistance throughout the preparation and publication of this book.

Carlos Miguel Rios-González
Facultad de Ciencias Médicas,
Universidad Nacional de Caaguazu,
Coronel Oviedo, Paraguay

Section 1

Introduction

Chapter 1

Introductory Chapter: Transgender Health - Advances and New Perspectives

Carlos Miguel Rios-González

1. Introduction

Transvestites, transsexuals, and transgender (Trans) people require specific particularities regarding their health care. That is why it is important to know and understand these needs in order to provide them with adequate and quality health care [1, 2].

The recognition of gender identity as a fundamental human right, the State must guarantee, in the field of health, that all health benefits are contemplated in the law of each country. Then, recognizing people as active subjects of law, especially in relation to personal decisions, such as self-perception of gender and body modifications, care will be provided according to specific needs [3].

Respect without prejudice and without discrimination must be valued in policies as a basis for the humanization, promotion, protection, care, and health care of Trans people [4]. In this way, facing all types of discrimination and social exclusion implies promoting the construction of citizenship and, at the same time, requires expanding the participation of health teams as mobilizers of defense, the right to health, and sexual and reproductive rights as a fundamental component of the health of al [5–7].

2. Health in Trans people

Despite the fact that this group constitutes a quantitatively and qualitatively relevant social group in our country, sexual orientation and gender identity are not included in most national health statistics and studies, so little is known about the specific needs, problems, and health inequalities of the Trans population around the world [8].

Despite the fact that in many countries the legislation protects the right to non-discrimination and, more specifically, to that based on sex and sexual orientation, as well as the right to life, liberty, and security of the LGBT community, many National and international organizations have highlighted the existence of numerous incidents of discrimination and violence against these people throughout the world, as well as episodes of discrimination from health services [9, 10].

Although the scientific evidence is still limited, studies conducted in other settings suggest that LGBT people face inequities in health and, compared to the heterosexual population, this group has a higher prevalence of certain health problems related

IntechOpen

to social stigma and denial of their rights. The lack of personal, family, and social acceptance in relation to non-normative sexual orientation and gender identity can affect the mental health and the safety and well-being of Trans people [11, 12].

The discrimination suffered by these people has been associated with high rates of psychiatric illness, substance abuse, suicide, and victimization. These negative experiences can produce lasting psychosocial consequences both in the people who suffer them directly and in the rest of the group. Undoubtedly, prejudice and hatred towards this group play a crucial role in this health problem, added to the emotional, psychological, and physical damage caused by stigmatization, isolation, humiliation, harassment, and verbal and physical [13].

Usually, the specific health needs of the Trans population are insufficiently known or even ignored by health authorities and health professionals. According to the limited literature available, this population has higher rates of mental health disorders, such as depression, anxiety, and suicide, as well as substance abuse, such as tobacco, alcohol, and other recreational drugs. The approach to this matter is complex since within each identity there are different problems [14].

Likewise, the health needs and problems of Trans people are different throughout the life cycle: for example, during adolescence and early youth, there is a greater risk of suicide and being homeless. In adulthood, the Trans population has higher rates of tobacco, alcohol, and drug abuse, and in old age, they often face other health barriers due to social isolation and lack of culturally competent health and social services [15].

In order to guarantee that Trans can enjoy a long and disease-free life, it is necessary to eliminate the health inequalities of this group. This requires a specific approach from the services and administrations in charge of public health, as well as specific health care, which contains a gender and human rights perspective [13, 15].

The benefits of improving their health and reducing these inequities include reduced health costs from avoidable health problems, increased longevity and well-being, both physical and psychological, and, as a positive externality, increased social welfare, and creative capacity, reducing inequalities in access to the labor market and increasing labor productivity [16].

Although there are several advances in terms of regulations and acceptance, there are still several barriers, to improve the quality of life of this population.

3. Conclusion

Any action aimed at addressing the health of Trans people must be carried out from a model that has a gender perspective, human rights, and respect for diversity, with the participation of the LGBT+ community, based on the principles of voluntariness and self-definition of people who agree to participate and respecting the privacy and confidentiality that these data require, without arbitrary interference in their private life.

Conflict of interest

The authors declare no conflict of interest.

Author details

Carlos Miguel Rios-González[1,2]

1 Faculty of Medical Sciences, National University of Caaguazu, Colonel, Oviedo, Paraguay

2 Ministry of Public Health and Social Welfare, National Institute of Health, Asunción, Paraguay

*Address all correspondence to: carlosmigue_rios@live.com

References

[1] De La Guardia Gutiérrez MA, Ruvalcaba Ledezma JC. La salud y sus determinantes, promoción de la salud y educación sanitaria. JONNPR. 2020;**5**(1):81-90

[2] World Health Organization. Glossary of Health Promotion Terms. Geneva: WHO; 2001. Available from: https://apps.who.int/iris/bitstream/handle/10665/67246/WHO_HPR_HEP_98.1_spa.pdf;jsessionid=F1A51668C6D78085735778F0DA17BFD0?sequence=1

[3] Organización Mundial de la Salud. Salud en las Américas. Capítulo 2 Determinantes e Inequidades en Salud. Ginebra: OMS; 2012. Available from: https://www.paho.org/salud-en-las-americas-2012/index.php?option=com_docman&view=download&category_slug=sa-2012-volumen-regional-18&alias=163-capitulo-2-determinantes-e-inequidades-salud-163&Itemid=231&lang=en

[4] World Health Organization. Commission on Social Determinants of Health. Redress Inequalities in a Generation. Final Report. Geneva: WHO/PAHO; 2008. Available from: https://www.paho.org/mex/index.php?option=com_docman&view=document&layout=default&alias=368-comision-sobre-determinantes-sociales-de-la-salud-resumen-analitico-del-2008-final-report&category_slug=equity-in-health&Itemid=493

[5] Braveman P, Egerter S, Williams DR. The social determinants of health: Coming of age. Annual Review of Public Health. 2011;**32**:381-398

[6] Kickbusch I. The political determinants of health—10 years on. BMJ. 2015;**350**

[7] Dawes DE. The Political Determinants of Health. Baltimore, Maryland, United States: Johns Hopkins University Press; 2020

[8] Tan KK, Schmidt JM, Ellis SJ, Veale JF. Mental health of trans and gender diverse people in Aotearoa/New Zealand: A review of the social determinants of inequities. New Zealand Journal of Psychology. 2019;**48**(2):64-72

[9] Restar A, Jin H, Operario D. Gender-inclusive and gender-specific approaches in trans health research. Transgender Health. 2021;**6**(5):235-239

[10] Ortiz-Martínez Y, Ríos-González CM. Need for more research on and health interventions for transgender people. Sexual Health. 2017;**14**(2):196-197

[11] De Benedictis-Serrano GA, Rios-González CM. The LGBT community and HIV: An incorrect medical judgment. Travel Medicine and Infectious Disease. 2018;**25**:18-19

[12] Suess SA. Trans health care from a depathologization and human rights perspective. Public Health Reviews. 2020;**41**(1):1-17

[13] T'Sjoen G, Arcelus J, De Vries AL, Fisher AD, Nieder TO, Özer M, et al. European Society for Sexual Medicine position statement "assessment and hormonal management in adolescent and adult trans people, with attention for sexual function and satisfaction". The Journal of Sexual Medicine. 2020;**17**(4):570-584

[14] Bell J, Purkey E. Trans individuals' experiences in primary care. Canadian Family Physician. 2019;**65**(4):e147-e154

[15] Zeeman L, Sherriff N, Browne K, McGlynn N, Mirandola M, Gios L, et al. A review of lesbian, gay, bisexual, trans and intersex (LGBTI) health and healthcare inequalities. European Journal of Public Health. 2019;**29**(5):974-980

[16] Daly A, Champion JD. Creating inclusive health care environments: Health care stories from the trans population. Journal of the American Association of Nurse Practitioners. 2021;**33**(6):451-458

Section 2

Social Determinants of Health

Chapter 2

Transfeminine Bodies: Survival and Resilience Experiences in Brazil

Silvana de Souza Nascimento and Luz Gonçalves Brito

Abstract

This article aims to provide the results of anthropological research in Brazil regarding how trans and transvestites have survived in a country that is world-ranked in transfeminicide and how they find ways of resistance and resilience through support and care from networks to public health policies. The methodology used in the research was based on a multisited ethnography, through fieldwork and qualitative interviews, in two different regions: the metropolitan area of João Pessoa, in the state of Paraíba, in the Northeast, and the metropolis of São Paulo, in the Southeast. Using an intersectional perspective, the results show an increase in risks and vulnerabilities by black transfeminine people, mostly those who work in prostitution, because they do not have access to public health systems and have informally produced their care strategies based on local knowledge about the body, health, hormonal therapy, and so forth.

Keywords: transfeminine people, Brazil, care, vulnerability, ethnography

1. Introduction

Lilith went to the basic health unit near her home in a big city of Brazil. She thought she had HIV and she wanted to make sure. Lilith was a middle class trans woman in process of social and hormonal transition. She studied social science at the university. Although she was not a sex worker, she had had unsafe sex, due to her extreme emotional vulnerability. She arrived at the basic health unit, watching her steps, unsecure about her appearance, even though she wore a mask, which hid her sparse laser-removed facial hair. There was an enormous line, and she asked someone if she could use the stairs. "Are you going to the infectious disease department, sir?" said out loud the ugly men in the front desk. He disrespected her twofold, misgendering her and exposing a presumed health status. She reached the stairs, thorn inside. While she was waiting in the line to schedule her appointment with the doctor, a white man, who was working in the reform of the windows in the public health center, noticed she was trans. He looked at her with creepy eyes, approached her, almost touching her, invading her personal space. Without any words, he was suggesting sex. Lilith was feeling terrible with her silent social suffering. She left the place, heading to the bakery. While she was paying for the cheese bread, a Black woman who was homeless came into the place and asked her for money. She could not help at that moment. Angry, the woman said: "You are just a boy who sits on cocks," and left. When Lilith arrived home, with all the transphobic situations returning over and over in her head, she looked at the windows of her room on the 10th floor. She thought it would be a final solution for her social suffering. She took out her clothes of her heavy body, stepped to the rampart, with anxious breath. She could not even feel the air. She imagined her monstruous armor floating in the direction of the morning blue sky. But she returned to the basic health unit, talked to the manager, and decided to report the harasser to the police. The women's bureau was not prepared to register cases like hers, not only because she was trans (the cops subtly laughed at her and one female cop was not sure if her case should be investigated there), but also because sexual harassment is naturalized in Brazil, even by the police, whose scope of action usually prioritizes domestic violence.

Social suffering, as Kleinman *et al.* [1] defined, is an important category of analysis when it comes to the experience of trans women and transvestites in Brazil.[1] The narrative above situates the evident and subtle social suffering, which is part of the lived experience of trans people in Brazil. The allegoric narrative contains some modalities of the structural violence experienced by a trans woman in process of social transition in the country. Such a structural violence involves misgendering, emotional and psychological abuse, sexual harassment, discrimination, misogyny, difficulties in accessing health services. The narrative is the composite picture that summarizes samples of oral information and written texts of transgender women gathered by means of ethnographic interviews during 15 years of research. Nevertheless, the situations experienced by a trans person are not merely personal problems, but rather social problems, which are experienced personally and aggravated by the different layers of intersectionality. A poor Black transvestite woman who does not have access to privileged spaces of knowledge production, such as a university, experiences other forms of oppression and violence, even though the main modalities of discrimination affect most trans women.

Along the narrative, the social problems are experienced as personal and intimate discomfort, anger and hate, leading to a sense of unease and bodily sensations of desperation, sadness, and hopelessness. Although such an experience could seem extremely particular, if we consider the wide set of research on the transgender experience in Euro-American societies, we will find that suicide ideation and trials are more common among trans people than among cisgender population [2]. We understand that such a prominent reality is a result of transphobia—the culturally shared hate discourses and structural violence by a certain society in detriment of trans people—and not a correlate fact relative to a supposedly inherently problematic identity [3].

We understand that most of the mental health issues experienced by transgender people are deep and intimate impacts of the sociological problem of transphobia. The core of transphobia is a naturalized, socially tolerated, and still unpunished violence against trans people (transgender men, transgender women, nonbinary people, and transvestites). In a country where transfeminicide exceeds all the rates in comparison to other nations [4–7], it is not surprising that trans people, and specifically transgender women and transvestites, need to face huge problems whose origins certainly are not a particular mental disease or an individual nonconformity.

[1] Alongside this text, we use trans women as an umbrella term that includes transgender women and Transexual women. Usually, the term trans is also used to encompass a set of diverse identities, such as non-binary and gender-non-confirming people.

In the context of this culturally shared hate, the cycles of violence faced by trans women and transvestites have been reiterated like a precise sociological pattern. The revelation of the transgender identity is frequently followed by parental alienation, abandonment, truancy, and—due to marginalization, exclusion, social hostility, and the lack of formation and social support—compulsory sex work, which often begins in the early adolescence. The dynamics of social vulnerabilities experienced by the population of trans women and transvestites in Brazil also impact their access to public health services.

In the face of adverse circumstances, trans women and transvestites create their own strategies of resilience through their own support and care networks. Interestingly, trans women and transvestites who work as sex workers declare that the experience of prostitution enables resilient ways of life, through which care networks and affective bonds are built [8–14].

This article will explore how trans women and transvestites have built their networks in order to survive in such a difficult social environment caused by the structural violence of transphobia. First, we delineate an overview of trans health in Brazil. The other two topics present ethnographic experience in the metropolitan area of João Pessoa, state of Paraíba, in the Northeast, and in the metropolis of São Paulo, situated in the Southeast. We conclude suggesting an analogy between the "Brazilian racism" explored by Lelia Gonzalez [15] and the "Brazilian transphobia." We also suggest that transvestites and trans women construct a lived knowledge on their own bodies as an important form of resistance.

2. Methodology

Since 2009, Professor Silvana de Souza Nascimento has coordinated ethnographic research regarding trans women and transvestites who work as sex workers in the Northeast and Southeast. First, in the Northeast region of the state of Paraíba, the fieldwork was done at one peripheral place, on the margins of a federal road, where transvestites from rural and Indigenous areas live, circulate, and work on the local sex markets. The aim of this primary research, between 2009 and 2012, was to understand how this population occupied and mobilized the territory. Two other circuits beyond prostitution were identified: the LGBTQIA+ movements and the beauty contests.[2] We could observe that transvestites and trans women who were sex workers at the contryside of Paraíba have a lifestyle translated on the road as an interstitial space, in its metaphorical and literal meaning, constituted on the borders of metropolitan regions. They circulate in small and medium-sized cities, relatively close to the main centers, whose strategic locality allows for a great circulation of people, vehicles, information, and networks of relations [12].

Research conducted in Paraíba followed the ethnographic method, including fieldwork, 15 interviews, and production of photographs. The ethnographic perspective is the theoretical base of our reflections, which are drawn upon the experience and the lived knowledge of our interlocutors.

[2] The first research, "Variations of the feminine: dialogue between gender, city and transexualities", funded by CNPQ, included the participation of young undergraduate researchers at the Federal University of Paraíba: Lívia Freire, Verônica Guerra, Luzicleide Bernardo and Thiago Oliveira, who are currently Masters or Phd students of Anthropology at different universities. Paulo Rossi, a photographer and sociologist, also participated.

> *The ethnographic theory aims to elaborate a model of comprehension of any social object (language, magic, politics) that, even though being produced in a particular context, may work as a matrix of intelligibility in other contexts (...) The ethnographic theory proceeds like the savage thought: takes the very much concrete elements collected in the fieldwork and articulates them in a little bit more abstract propositions, giving intelligibility to the happenings and the world. ([16], p. 460).*

In 2014, after her move to the University of São Paulo, Professor Silvana Nascimento began to research in São Paulo city. A new research project was developed, from 2015 to 2017.[3] The aim of the project was to comprehend the forms of urbanity by means of the transits and mobilities of trans women and transvestites in three regions of the country: in the metropolitan region of João Pessoa, Northeast; in the city of São Paulo, Southeast, specifically, the Butantã area; and in the triple Amazonic frontier, in the region of Alto Solimões, at the North, between the cities of Letícia (Colombia), Tabatinga (Brazil), and Santa Rosa (Peru). This text concerns only the two first regions mentioned above because the ethnographic data are more structured.

In São Paulo, research was conducted, mainly, at the spaces of prostitution in the Butantã area, near Cidade Universitária, where the biggest campus of the University of São Paulo is situated. During our interviews, in partnership with the Defensoria Pública do Estado de São Paulo and the Service of Specialized Assistance STD/SIDA of Butantã, we dispensed informative leaflets on the rights of sex workers and gender violence, besides condoms.

By means of a multisited ethnography, drawing upon the notion of sharing as the condition for a certain anthropological project, this ethnography is informed by transfeminism, putafeminismo, by the demands of trans movements, and by the wide knowledge produced by trans researchers ([6, 17–24], among many others).

3. Trans health in Brazil

The recognition of "trans" as a socially visible identity is inherently tied to the public health policies that included the population of trans people. Hand in hand with those policies, the recognition of gender identity of trans people was widely divulgated for health providers in the context of SUS, the Brazilian national public health system. An important identity policy was the recognition of the social name. The main health policies are the processes of gender affirmation, such as sex reassignment surgery and other related body transformations, provided by a dozen hospitals in the country. The pioneers were Hospital de Clínicas (Porto Alegre-Rio Grande do Sul); Hospital das Clínicas (Goiânia-Goiás); Hospital de Clínicas

[3] The research entitled "Trans-cities: experiences among people, frontiers and places" was funded by Fundação de Amparo à Pesquisa do Estado de S. Paulo (Fapesp) and Pró-Reitoria de Pesquisa of the University of São Paulo (Edital Novos Docentes). The following undergraduate students at USP participated: Alexandre Martins, Beatriz Rossi, Maria Iachinski Natália Corazza, Sabrina Damaceno e Lucas Vechi. And included the participation of the following graduate students of Anthropology: Veronica Guerra (Universidade Federal da Pernambuco/UFPE), Thiago de Lima Oliveira (USP), Luiza Lima (USP) e Letizia Patriarca (USP). Flávia Melo, Professor of Anthropology of UFAM (Federal Universidade of Amazonas) and José Miguel Olivar Nieto, researcher of the Group of Gender Studies Pagu/UNICAMP (Universidade Estadual de Campinas).

(Recife-Pernambuco); Hospital Universitário Pedro Ernesto (Rio de Janeiro-Rio de Janeiro); e Hospital das Clínicas (São Paulo-São Paulo).

"Transexualizer process" regards the set of specialized services offered to trans people as a public health service. It encompasses endocrinological follow-up, psychological and social support, and surgeries. The transexualizer process was first stablished in 2008 by the Ministry of Health by means of Portaria 1707 and Portaria 457.[4] In 2013, the "transexualizer process" was expanded and included as part of the National Policy of LGBT Integral Health. According to Cardoso ([25]: 6), the main goal of the National Policy of LGBT Integral Health is "promoting the integral health of lesbians, gays, bisexual people, and trans people, and eliminating discrimination and institutional prejudice, as well as the reduction of inequalities and consolidation of SUS as universal, integral and equitable."

More recently, family health facilities began to offer basic assistance to trans people, regardless of their participation on the "transexualizer process" of SUS. This is remarkable because these "ambulatórios" propose another perspective on transgender health. On the one hand, they propose a non-pathologizing practice, avoiding the confinement of identities by the diagnosis of gender dysphoria.[5] On the other hand, they do not prevent gender nonconforming people and nonbinary people to access services of hormone therapy or other relative therapeutic processes. The notion of a "true transsexual" is abandoned, favoring self-determination of identity and including people who would not fit the criteria of a psychiatric diagnosis.

Even though the "ambulatórios" are, indeed, more inclusive than the biggest hospitals of reference, there is a parcel of trans population who still face more difficulties in accessing health services: the poor Black transvestites. In fact, gender, class, and race as social markers of difference overlap, engendering forms of discrimination, which are increased and shifted depending on how these social markers are embodied and perceived in social relations. Rego [7] suggested that the state plays an important role in the extermination of the abject bodies, particularly trans, Black, and poor people. The difficulties of poor and Black trans people in being truly included and welcome at public health spaces are the extension of their marginalization of social life as a whole. According to Rego, "afronecrotransphobia is a politics of symbolic and actual extermination of Black trans people; politics that affect living and take away life" ([7], p. 179) Afronecrotransphobia is rooted in the social hierarchy of bodies who deserve to live and others who are not "grievable."

These different forms of violence, according to Snorton [26], clearly reveal the failures of the promise made by the state and its technique of production of a "racialized gender." In other words, it is necessary to investigate the articulation between gender and race in order to understand the specific form of violence against trans people and transvestites. Such a violence denunciates the grammar of a genocide state and demonstrates the construction of a continuous state of emergency for this population. "There is no absolute difference between the importance of Black lives and trans lives under the sign of the racialized gender" ([26], p. 13).

We understand that the visibility of trans identities in Brazil is largely tied to the institutionalization of public health services for trans people. Nevertheless, trans visibility in Brazil is due more to the social action of Black transvestites by means of the trans movement. Trans woman and transvestites, especially the Black ones, have always been very important for the activism in Brazil, likely Marsha P. Johnson and

---

[4] Portaria is an official document signed by a state leadership in Brazil.

[5] See International Classification of Deseases 11th: https://icd.who.int/en.

Sylvia Rivera during the sixties in the Gay Liberation Front. Fernanda Benvenutty, for example, a transvestite who became an important political leadership is well recognized, and her photograph can be seen in the posters of the campaign for the social name, which are affixed to the walls at the public hospitals all around the country.[6]

4. The experience of the streets

The activist Fernanda Benvenutty (1962–2020), one of our interlocutors who followed our work in Paraíba, was a Black transvestite. She was born in a small city of Paraíba and participated in the trans movement, locally and nationally. Fernanda had an important trajectory in the field of trans health, participating in national and regional councils. She also participated in the process of foundation of ABGLT and ANTRA (National Association of Transsexuals and Transvestites), with Keyla Sympson, another Black transvestite. When she was a member of CNS (National Health Council), which established the national politics of health at that time, she became a protagonist of the campaign for the social name of transvestites and transexuals in the realm of SUS. The campaign included, specially, the distribution of posters with images of transvestites and trans women to the health facilities and hospitals. It aimed to inform about the existence of the legitimacy of the social name, defending the guaranteed use of the social name as part of the citizenship for transexuals and transvestites.

Locally, in Paraíba, Fernanda was one of the founders of ASTRAPA (Association of Transvestites and Transexual of Paraíba). Together with Movimento do Espírito Lilás (gay movement) and Grupo de Mulheres Lésbicas e Bissexuais Maria Quitéria, Fernanda organized numberless seminars, debates, meetings and proposed public policies for the local and regional governments. In 2017, she collaborated with the creation of the Ambulatório de Saúde Integral Travestis e Transexuais da Paraíba.[7]

Fernanda was not only an activist of the LGBTQIA+ movement. She was a nurse technician who worked for more than 20 years at a public maternity hospital, where she participated in hundreds of childbirth processes. She also worked at a psychiatric hospital. Her experience in the field of public health made her well known and respected not only by the professionals, but also by the users of the hospitals. Thus, through her political and professional action, she built a network of care and affection beyond her biological and familiar circle. In the region she lived, she founded a *Samba School* (Unidos do Roger), which became a space of solidarity and possibilities for people who had dissident gender identities and sexual orientations. Consequently, her house was the main space for the *Samba School* and a gathering place for LGBTQIA+. Fernanda was the leader of the *Samba School*, and she took care of everybody as a family united by affection and care, with her attentive, rigid, and controlling maternity.

As the director of ASTRAPA, Fernanda contributed to the aforementioned research, participating in projects against transphobia at the University of Paraíba. She also participated in the photographic exhibition "Variations of the Feminine: poetics of the trans universe," in 2010 and 2011, whose aim was to create the visibility of non-exoticizing images of trans women, transvestites, and effeminate homosexuals that could reveal details, feeling, and gestures, which could touch the sensibility of

6 https://bvsms.saude.gov.br/bvs/cartazes/nome_social_sus.pdf.

7 The Ambulatório TT of Paraíba offers services for the specialized care of trans people by a multiprofissional team, including psychologist, psychiatrist, social worker, nurse, gynecologist, and urologist.

the public. During the exhibition, one room excelled: a photographic essay created by the anthropologist Verônica Guerra [27], the register of a 19-year-old Black transvestite, Márcia, who had been killed recently. Márcia was born in the rural area of Paraíba and worked as a prostitute since early age, mainly on the federal road of the North Litoral region.[8] Nevertheless, aiming to increase her income, invited by a more experienced transvestite, she decided to move to Recife, biggest city of the state of Pernambuco, where the levels of urban violence are very much higher. Thus, shortly after her moving to Recife, Márcia was brutally assassinated on the street. There are rumors that she was trying to help a colleague who was being violated, and Márcia was shot. Her case was not even reported officially as transfeminicide, and her social name was not respected in her death certification.

Unfortunately, this tragic history is a reality for trans women and transvestites raised by poor families in vulnerable situations, especially for those who work in the sex markets. They leave their original places, moving to bigger cities where they can achieve better conditions of life and income. The circulation by different cities in Brazil and abroad is part of the dynamics of the sex markets, but it also suggests a lifestyle: a constant movement of seeking for oneself, for one's own body and the desired gender, the scape from the violence of transphobia and racism, from cisheteronormativity. A mobility that brings financial support in order to survive and obtain the necessary body interventions (hormone therapy, surgeries, cosmetics, clothes, and so forth). It is a journey toward a possible and safe future, where one could live and guarantee the rights of citizenship.

> *They move between cities and model themselves in the fabric of temporary experiences in places that offer them the possibilities for social and economic ascension and that, at the same time, are more likely to accept their ways of being, past and present, usually considered abject. ([28], p. 192)*

The death of Márcia adds to the statistics of transfeminicide. However, following the argument of Snorton, it is necessary to go beyond the obvious acknowledgement of the high rates of homicides of Black trans people, considering the loss of the subject, their memory, and their future.

> *The recurring practice of enumerating the assassinated people on the press and social media seems to coadunate with the logic of accumulation that structurates the racial capitalism, where the quantified abstraction of trans and Black deaths reveals the calculated value of trans and Black lives by means of the grammar of a state of doubt and deficit ([26], p. 10)*

Transvestites like Márcia circulate constantly by different cities. The mobility is facilitated by the existence of a federal road (BR 101) that connects different big cities. In these areas, they attend clients who are, mainly, truckers, travelers, and workers of the sugarcane plants. They meet at strategic points, such as gas stations, where there is a great circulation of people and money. Those who live in João Pessoa, circulate by the beaches, on medium and high-class regions, but also Downtown, an impoverished region.

[8] The North Litoral of Paraíba is a microrregion encompassing 11 small municipalities, which are part of the Metropolitan Region of João Pessoa. This region also encompasses other contiguous areas, near the main city, João Pessoa, with small and medium scale cities (up to 70 hundred inhabitants).

The main work in the sex markets is street prostitution and work at websites that offer sexual services (presential or virtual meetings by means of live cams). The latter increased in the last years, especially during the COVID-19 pandemic in 2020. Most clients are cisgender men who identify as straights. Often, they are married or maintain stable relationships. They vary in age, class, and occupation. Nevertheless, depending on the city or territory where the prostitutes work, there are meaningful economic differences and the clients' profile and prices shift.

According to ANTRA, more than 90% of the transfeminine population in Brazil worked or has worked as sex workers, at least once in the lifetime. Besides being a source of income, the prostitution allows for the creation of networks of affection, support, and care. The prostitution is also a space—be it the streets, houses, or hostels—where a feminine identity is constructed. The prostitution houses are also places of sociability and, usually, are governed by older or more experienced transvestites and trans women, who are called "madrinhas" or "mothers" [9, 14, 29]. These entanglements of economic relations and affection relations [30] also recreate kinship and friendship relations.

According to Manuel Roberto Escobar [31], the trans body can be understood as a baroque body whose movements go beyond its own objectives, escaping from the homogeneity of the capitalist *ethos*. Escobar suggests that the trans body is pure excess of meaning, which is transformed by means of esthetic, surgical, and pharmacological interventions. The trans body is attentive to all details, ornaments, and gestures that are revealed or occulted. They overflow the frontiers, and their transformations affect their surrounding worlds, modifying the spaces through which they move.

In Paraíba, the interlocutors of research were young transvestites who were raised in the region and kept their relations, more or less hostile, with their families and places of origin. Most of them wanted to move to other city and obtain more income with sex work, in order to pursue their body transformations more adequately. In São Paulo, the biggest Brazilian metropolis, the reality is quite different.

With more than 12 million inhabitants, São Paulo receives hundreds of transvestites and trans women from different regions of Brazil and also from Latin America. The central region of the city is well known for the services of prostitution, consumption, and sociability. Besides Downtown, a place with touristic and national projection, other localities are important. Among them, the region of Butantã is remarkable. Situated in the West Zone of São Paulo, near USP main campus, Butantã is inhabited by 5400 people and, historically, is an area of great circulation of people, alternating commercial and residential streets.

During our fieldwork, we talked to more than 40 transvestites and trans women, whose age varied from 16 to 40 years old. They were born mainly in the North and Northeast of Brazil, in the cities such as Manaus (Amazonas), Belém (Pará), Natal (Rio Grande do Norte), Recife (Pernambuco), and Fortaleza (Ceará). Many tranvestites and trans women stay shortly, from 1 week up to 6 months, especially the young. The older ones, 25 years old or more, stay longer, from 5 to 15 years, but they also create intense mobility, moving to other cities and countries. These people rarely settle in a single territory, especially the young ones. Often, they live in collective residences, where they share their lives with other transvestites from the same region, their friends.

The daily reality of trans women and transvestites from North and Northeast is coming to São Paulo, where they work as prostitutes. Regardless of their origin, they have the same project of social mobility: making money through sex work, accessing a network of esthetic consumption, making their bodies more feminine by means of hormonal and surgical interventions. During our fieldwork, we collected many reports of body transformation, particularly hormonal therapy experiences, with or without medical follow-up, and use of industrial silicone for body feminization.

Industrial silicone, despite its risks to health, has still been used to modify the body because the prices are lower than surgeries. Due to the insufficiency of SUS in providing surgeries and a long line in which many trans people wait for their turn, many transvestites and trans women search for liquid silicone, in order to achieve shortly the desired ideal body. However, the substance is not indicated for human application. It is used for machine lubrication, automobiles, and civil construction, causing serious consequences in the human bodies [32]. According to the Muriel Project, in Brazil, there is a preference for the injection of SLI on the buttocks, hips, and thighs because the prosthesis for the breasts became more accessible in the private health systems where, often, these women pay for the plastic surgery instead of waiting for the slow process of SUS.

> *The use of SLI can bring the fast body transformations, representing the valuing of a capital of the body. It means that an ideal body also brings more clients and value. On the other hand, some people who use SLI or undergo other procedures may increase their workload in the sexual market in order to enable for its payment, also increasing the risk for HIV infection because they have worse conditions of negotiation with clients, becoming more vulnerable to unprotected practices ([32], p. 10).*

Those trans women and transvestites who work as sex workers often need fast transformations and enhancements of their bodies. Therefore, they cannot wait for the long process of transformation enabled by the hormone therapy. Some medications such as estradiol enantate/algestone acetophenide (Perlutan®) are well known by the trans community for its quick effects of breasts and buttocks augmentation and general feminization of the body due to liquid retention. Trans women and transvestites who use this injection of estradiol anecdotally report the fast reversion of the augmentation when they stop its continuous use.

In the region of Butantã, there is a basic health center, binding to the University of São Paulo, where trans people are welcome to access some public health services. In the same region, there is also a center of reference for HIV,[9] where prevention agents act. Nevertheless, the great challenge is to include sex workers in this health spaces. During our fieldwork, many trans women and transvestites told us that the opening hours are reduced, and they cannot go there early morning because they work all night long. They also reported a disrespect for their correct pronouns at different kinds of private and public services, even if they do have their new documents. They also distrust the treatment they will receive by health providers because their experiences of transphobia and racism are numberless.

Despite all difficulties, Fernanda, a white trans woman born in Fortaleza (Ceará, Northeast), works as prevention agent daily with the prostitutes. She dispenses condoms and lubrication gel, talking to them about forms of preventions and health care. Furthermore, she often hosts other transvestites and trans women who are experiencing situations of violence or working difficulties and sickness derived from the use

---

[9] Even though the official Brazilian statistics do not report the prevalence of HIV among trans women and transvestites, research suggests that they are the population most affected by the virus (ROCHA, ABM; BARROS, CRS; PRADO, I.; BASTOS, F. I.; VERAS, MA. HIV continuum of care among trans women and travestis living in São Paulo, Brazil. *Revista de Saúde Pública*, v. 54, 54:118, 2020).

of industrial silicone. Like Fernanda of Paraíba, the house of Fernanda of São Paulo is also a place where webs of affection, mutual help, and solidarity are weaved. Both work in the field of health, and through this experience, they also support others who need their care. After long years working as a prostitute, Fernanda of São Paulo became an autonomous entrepreneur. She owns a sewing atelier where she creates and sells clothes. The atelier is her main source of income. "Each day is a step we make onward."

Even though we have not done fieldwork during the COVID-19 pandemic, we visited twice the territory of Butantã. Transvestites and trans women reported that, despite the risks, they were unable to follow social distancing protocols because they needed to maintain their work, circulating by different regions and cities. They also needed to avoid face masks most of the time in order to attract their clients. At this territory of prostitution, it seems there was a private security control of their circulation, especially in front of business buildings where they cannot neither stay nor stop for their clients in the cars. Before the pandemic, there was a circulation of pedestrians and cars, but today the streets are desert. Only transvestites and trans women are present. The empty space also increased the vulnerability and risk of violence.

Thus, amid numberless situations of violence and transphobia, working as sex workers enables economic and social alternatives, even though trans women and transvestites are more vulnerable in the streets. However, many think the risks are worthy. Others think the streets engender circumstances of moral, sexual, physical, and gender violence.

5. Conclusion

An important question deeply explored by transfeminist intellectuals like Amara Moira and Megg Rayara Oliveira [23, 33] concerns the stereotypical image of transvestites always seen with a bias of sexualization, bodies subject to violation. This image is related to the sexualized figure of Brazilian Black women, the *mulata*. Lélia Gonzalez [15] discussed that the idea of *mulata* is a historic unfolding of the figure of *mucama*, the domestic enslaved woman who worked for the patriarchal white family and who suffered from numberless violations. During carnival, the image of the *mulata* is exalted at the samba parade by national and international mass media. *Mulata* is an emblematic figure on the postal cards of Brazilian tourism and on TV advertising. Thus, during the parades of *Samba Schools*, *mulatas* are recognized, demonstrating her artistic gifts through her dance and beautiful, shining bodies. However, according to Gonzalez [15], the day after the parade she returns to the world of the house, becoming again a maid who lives in precarious conditions and who are explored as cheap workforce and sexual object. This is what Gonzalez [15] calls "Brazilian racism."

Similarly, at the catwalk of the streets, transvestites parade their splendid wishful bodies and attract men looking for sex and affection. There, at the sidewalks, they weave webs of solidarity among friends and colleagues, strive for survival, and learn local knowledge on hormones, men, sexual relations, prevention, safety, and so forth. Nevertheless, the same territory presents serious risks because they are exposed to numberless forms of transphobic and racist violence. It is no coincidence that Brazil is ranked as the most dangerous place to trans people, with enormous rates of transfeminicide, but at the same time one of the countries where transvestite pornography is extremely consumed. Many narratives of violence at public spaces, perpetuated by men (cops, clients, partners, security guards) against trans women and transvestites, particularly the Black ones, reveal common situations where there is a clear trial of masculine domination, demonstration of authority and humiliation. Drawing inspiration upon the reflections of Lélia Gonzalez, we may call this process "Brazilian transphobia": the place of simultaneous desire and rejection of people who contest the patriarchal cisnormativities overlapped by the Whiteness.

Since the beginning of 2000, trans movements have claimed strongly for the construction of public policies on the realm of health, education, and work. Even though there are important milestones—such as the recognition of social name by public and private institutions, the right of changing birth documents, and the access to the transexualizer process of SUS—numberless events, situations, and practices of transphobia are still observed at public and private spaces, streets, schools, universities, workplaces, and so forth. The most vulnerable spaces for transvestites and trans women are the streets, where most of them work as sex workers. But paradoxically this occupation embraces them.

In this context of precarity, vulnerability, and gender violence, an important strategy of resistance is the lived knowledge regarding trans bodies, constructed by trans people. This lived knowledge is rooted in the experience of trans women and transvestites. The core tenet of such a knowledge is the experience with hormone therapies, a safe way to achieve body transformations. The exchange of this knowledge happens through different networks of care (forums on the Internet, collective residences, hostels, and streets).

Lived knowledge on their body transformations is a form of resistance because the structural transphobia implies subtle and open forms of discrimination against trans people. Therefore, trans women and transvestites share and apply this knowledge, in order to live fully and express their gender identities. The difficulties in accessing health services are counterbalanced by the lived knowledge on the transformations of the trans bodies. Although the medical community tends to validate academic knowledge, it is necessary to understand the experience of the lived body. If health providers are sufficiently humble to welcome their knowledge, trans people will probably feel more welcome. Evidently, trans women and transvestites, particularly the poorest ones, often trust on anecdotal and merely empirical reports of hormone use, shared by other trans people. There may be some incongruencies and disinformation, but scientific knowledge also fails sometimes. Nevertheless, it is important to recognize the relevance of the "savage thought"[10] that trans people create to express their experiences of their lived bodies. The repetition and patterns of hormone use are nothing but experiments, which lead to a form of knowledge, a lived knowledge.

The body transformations of trans people are not pathological. They can be understood as a human search for self-acceptance. Even though trans identities are not dependent on bodily transformations, body transformations are very important to many trans women and transvestites. Body transformations guarantee minimal social acceptance. Nevertheless, trans bodies are still seen as unintelligible because the normal bodies, according to the historical categories of normal and abject, are referenced by cisheteronormativity. The trend is that, with time and trans visibility and representativity, society will accept and expand the cultural constructs regarding trans people. Trans existences are embodied in multiple corporalities, which are never homogenized or pasteurized because trans identities extrapolate and implode the possibilities that the century considers acceptable or natural.

---

[10] Here, we borrowed the idea of Lévi-Strauss on the construction of a science of the concrete.
LÉVI-STRAUSS, Claude et al. *La pensée sauvage*. Paris: Plon, 1962.

Acknowledgement

This study was financed in part by the Coordenação de Aperfeiçoamento de Pessoal de Nível Superior - Brasil (CAPES) - Finance Code 001 and by CNPQ (Process 312677/2019-7).

Author details

Silvana de Souza Nascimento and Luz Gonçalves Brito*
Department of Anthropology, FFLCH - University of São Paulo (USP), Brazil

*Address all correspondence to: luzgoncalves@usp.br

References

[1] Kleinman A, Das V, Lock M, editors. Social Suffering. Un. Of California Press; 1997

[2] Silva RR, da Silva LA, de Souza MVL, da Silva MVG, das Neves MP, de Vargas D, et al. Estresse de minoria de gênero e seus efeitos na saúde mental como fator de risco para depressão em pessoas transgênero: Revisão da literatura. Research, Society and Development. 2021;**10**(3)

[3] Favero S. Pajubá-terapia: ensaios sobre a cisnorma. Porto Alegre: Nemesis Editora; 2020

[4] Carrara S, Vianna A. "Tá lá o corpo estendido no chão...": a violência letal contra travestis no município do Rio de Janeiro. Physis: revista de saúde coletiva. 2006;**16**:233-249

[5] Bento B. Brasil: país do transfeminicídio. Centro Latinio Americano em Sexualidade e Saúde (CLAM); 2014

[6] Gomes de Jesus J. Transfobia e crimes de ódio: Assassinatos de pessoas transgênero como genocídio. História Agora. 2014;**16**:101-123

[7] Rego YLP. Reflexões Sobre Afronecrotransfobia: Políticas de Extermínio na Periferia. Humanidades & Inovação. 2019;**6**(16):167-181

[8] Kulick D. Travesti – prostituição, sexo, gênero e cultura no Brasil. Rio de Janeiro: Fiocruz; 2008

[9] Patriarca L. Donas de casa, de prostituição: sobre as violências decorrentes da criminalização dos contextos destas práticas. Revista de Estudos Empíricos em Direito. 2019;**5**(3)

[10] Pelúcio L. Na noite nem todos os gatos são pardos. Notas sobre a prostituição travesti. Cadernos Pagu. 2005;**25**:217-248

[11] Pelúcio L. Abjeção e desejo: uma etnografia travesti sobre o modelo preventivo de aids. In: Tese (Doutorado) - Programa de Pós-Graduação em Ciências Sociais da Universidade Federal de São Carlos. 2007. p. 312p

[12] Nascimento S. Variações do feminino: circuitos do universo trans na Paraíba. Revista de Antropologia. 2014ª;**57**(2):377-411

[13] Nascimento S. Corpo-afeto, corpo-violência: experiências na prostituição de estrada na Paraíba. Revista Ártemis. 2014b;(18):1

[14] Sander VS e M. *Entre manuais e truques*: uma etnografia das redes do trabalho sexual entre travestis em Belo Horizonte. Dissertação de Mestrado em Antropologia Social, Unicamp. 2015

[15] Gonzalez L. Racismo e sexismo na cultura brasileira. Revista Ciências Sociais Hoje, Anpocs. 1984:223-244

[16] Goldman M. Os tambores dos mortos e os tambores dos vivos. Etnografia, antropologia e política em Ilhéus, Bahia. In: *Revista de Antropologia*. Vol. 46,n° 2. São Paulo: USP; 2003

[17] Almeida G. 'Homens trans': novos matizes na aquarela das masculinidades? Revista Estudos Feministas. 2012;**20**(2): 513-523

[18] Andrade L. Travestis na escola: assujeitamento e resistência à ordem normativa. Fortaleza: Doutorado em Educação, Universidade Federal do Ceará; 2012

[19] García Becerra A. Tacones, siliconas, hormonas y otras críticas al sistema sexo género. Feminismos y experiencias de transexuales y travestis. Revista Colombiana de Antropología. 2009;**2009**(1):119-146

[20] Lanz L. O corpo da ropa. A pessoa transgênera entre a transgressão e a conformidade com as normas de gênero. Curitiba: Disertación de Maestría en Sociología, Universidade Federal do Paraná; 2014

[21] Missé M, Coll-Planas G, editors. El género desordenado. Críticas en torno a la patologización de la transexualidad. Barcelona; Madrid: Egales; 2010

[22] Moira A. E se eu fosse puta. São Paulo: Hoo Editora; 2016

[23] Nery J. Viagem solitária: memórias de um transexual 30 anos depois. São Paulo: Leya; 2011

[24] Vergueiro V. Por infexões decoloniais de corpos e identidades de gênero inconformes: uma análise autoetnográfica da cisgeneridade como normatividade. Salvador: Dissertação de mestrado na área Multidisciplinar Cultura e Sociedade. Universidade Federal da Bahia; 2015

[25] Cardoso R. Anatomia do SUS: narrativas do cotidiano de uma formação em saúde coletiva. In: Trabalho de Conclusão de Residência, Residência Multiprofissional Integrada em Saúde Coletiva. UFRGS; 2021 [mimeo]

[26] Snorton R. Negra por los cuatro costados – una historia racial de la identidad trans. Barcelona: Bellaterra ediciones; 2017

[27] Guerra V. Sou salobra: travestilidade, lazer e sociabilidade no Litoral Norte da Paraíba. Dissertação de mestrado em Antropologia. Universidade Federal da Paraíba; 2015

[28] Nascimento S. Desire-cities: A transgender ethnography in the urban boundaries. Vibrant - Virtual Brazilian Anthropology. 2018;**15**

[29] Silva H. *Travesti:* a invenção do feminino. Rio de Janeiro: Relume-Dumará; 1993

[30] Zelizer V. Dinheiro, poder e sexo. Cadernos Pagu. 2009;(32) Campinas Jan/June

[31] Escobar MR. La politización del cuerpo: subjetividades *trans* em resistencia. Nómadas. 2013;**38**:133-149

[32] Pinto TB, Teiceira FB, Barros RB, et al. Silicone líquido industrial para transformar o corpo: prevalência e fatores associados ao seu uso entre travestis e mulheres transexuais em São Paulo, Brasil. Cadernos de Saúde Pública. 2017

[33] de Oliveira, Megg Rayara Gomes. Por que você não me abraça? Reflexões a respeito da invisibilização de travestis e mulheres transexuais no movimento social de negras e negros. Revista Sur 28, v.15, n.28, pp. 167-179, 2018.

Chapter 3

Public Policies Advances on Transgender People in Portugal

Dalia Costa and Miguel Miranda

Abstract

When rights are guaranteed through public policy, the probability of becoming *de facto* rights rather than just *de jure* rights is greatly increased. On the one hand, the conditions and mechanisms for its implementation are created or, at least, foreseen, and the conditions for effective access by all people to the rights in question are reviewed. This is the case of Portugal in promoting the rights of trans people, following a consolidated public policy on equality and gender (since 2007). The countries in Europe (European Union) have adopted different perspectives and paths ahead regarding the definition and implementation of comprehensive public policies for trans people. Previous studies about Portuguese case reveal that health, work, but also rights in the family and sexuality, are fragile domains, which place trans people in a situation of great vulnerability. Adopting a participatory methodology, the chapter presents the diversity in political and ideological positions and debates the obstacles in the process of public policy formulation to promote the integral well-being of trans people. The evaluation of the Portuguese case is useful for other political and social contexts, while it reveals the cornerstones of public policies advances on transgender persons, namely stereotypes and gender biases.

Keywords: gender identity, trans, self-determination, public policy, Portugal

1. Introduction

This chapter describes the process of advances in public policy, applied to the recognition of the right to gender identity and the sexual characteristics of people, including transgender. Portugal is the case study.

The Portuguese case is interesting because it has a recent democratic regime (since 1976) consolidated with the State's accession to the European Union (EU) in 1986. This social and political path shows a slow development until the 1990s focusing on the country's economic growth. This explains why it was only in the late 1990s that society began to wake up to plurality, including the uniqueness of people due to their gender identity.

Another fact that makes the Portuguese case interesting is that this period coincided with the resurgence of equality issues in the European context. Throughout the chapter, we demonstrate how Portugal aligned itself with other social contexts at the turn of the century. In the 1990s, the concept of gender entered the scientific lexicon. In addition, the pressure groups have also helped to make it part of the political

IntechOpen

agenda. These two elements are important for the process of construction of the right to gender self-determination, which culminated in the legislation of this right in 2018.

In an attempt to contribute to the in-depth knowledge of this process, we carried out a study with its main protagonists: deputies in the Portuguese parliament, who have the capacity and legitimacy for decision-making; social activists, with opportunities to emphasize the relevance of the right to self-determination of gender identity, specifically for transgender people; and social scientists who, in some cases, are also politicians or deputies and, in other cases, are also activists.

The study revealed the importance of external factors for deputies, such as voter expectations. It also revealed the importance of debate for the appropriation of concepts, questioning stereotypes in the public policies process production.

In the policy process analysis, we adopt the political pluralism, as the most suitable model for the analysis of a complex topic. This means that we are not going to analyze the content of the policy, but the policy production process, interviewing the main protagonists in that process.

In the first point of the chapter, we frame the theme. In the second, we describe the Portuguese context, to locate readers. We then present the study, highlighting its main results.

2. New perspectives on trans people

New perspectives on transgender people are relatively recent. The identification of transgender as an (autonomous) gender identity can be located in the paradigm shift generated from the conceptualization of gender. The ideological construction of a trans person began only after the appropriation of the gender concept. After that, the social problem construction process started, questioning how to deal with trans and how to answer to their expectations and needs, adapting public responses and their mechanisms. The next point follows this order.

2.1 A paradigm shift towards essentialist determinism

The concept of gender emerged from the feminist debate, chronologically identified with the second wave of this social, political and ideological movement, on the 1970s. Its operative dimension made it possible to deal with the 'anxieties of placing the issue of differences between the sexes on the social research agenda, removing it from the domain of biology'. At the same time that it was willing to 'orient its analysis to the historical and social conditions of production of beliefs and knowledge about the sexes and the legitimization of social divisions based on sex' [1].

In this way, the gender perspective allowed for an effective shift towards the differential Psychology of sexes approach, which explains differences between men and women, and towards Biology, which defines differences based on a nature determinism. Scientifically in the field of social sciences, and, later, politically, this can be considered 'an important transformation' [2] or, as the authors of this text consider it, a paradigmatic shift.

We consider this a paradigm shift for three main reasons. First, because it favored the emergence and subsequent imposition of another paradigm of interpretation of society and social relations in everyday life, replacing the paradigm of biology and psychology, both based on an interpretation of nature. Alternatively, the interpretation of the environment, the context or the social, encourages considering more factors in explaining the complexity of social relations.

Secondly, for giving to the scientific community and to the political community as well, specific concepts with a new meaning. Thus, thinking, describing and interpreting differences become possible through a concept, that of gender. Having a concept available, in turn, raises questions and drives away determinism. Among the questions were the extent and depth of social norms and expectations in shaping masculinities and femininities. Another issue linked to this was the weight of social structures on individuals, constraining their self-determination. The questioning of patriarchal social norms and broad expectations of performance of a social role defined by the sex of individuals at birth became easier.

Being born a man or a woman makes a difference and accentuates a determinism that is difficult to change, especially by common sense. It is very different to admit that one is born with a reproductive physiological system, but that we become men or women, through the induction of social processes, as Simone de Beauvoir had stated in her famous book (published in 1949).

It is very different because it opens up the concept of identity and establishes the importance of culture and the action of social structures on subjects. Thirdly, we believe that this is a paradigm shift because it has transformed the way of interpreting people, their relationships and the ways in which societies are organized around the way they interpret people. Gender is not determined but socially constructed; therefore, societies have a transforming capacity to change the subordination of the feminine to the masculine [3]. Gender, by ceasing to be something biologically determined, also ceased to be seen as something static, natural and immutable.

Considering that gender 'is not just about identity, not just work, not just power, not just sexuality, but all of this at the same time' [4], the complexity thickens. In this text, this complexity is addressed in relation to trans people who biologically have a male or female mark but who have a gender identity that does not coincide with that mark and socially impose who they are.

Being trans is more than the affirmation of a gender identity because it involves social interactions, thus implying social structures and mechanisms to guarantee equality, rights and de facto, that is, in everyday life.

2.2 New perspectives based on what means to be trans

The interpretation of a trans person began by being based on the most available and dominant model: the biological. Thus, the dimension of sexuality became the most relevant.

Western scientific communities have developed two relevant conceptual approaches: the concept of transsexuality and the concept of transgender. Transsexuality suggests a biomedical model, popularized in part by the North American contributions of John Money in the 1970s [5], and basically seeks to understand a situation in which the individual's gender contrasts with the physiological identification of sex.

The concept of transgender gained prominence from the 1990s onwards with the expansion of gender studies and the post-structuralist trend within the social sciences, distancing themselves from biomedical contributions. Authors such as Butler place the emphasis of their critical analysis on the binary gender system [6] that manages to associate biological characteristics with the sphere of social phenomena, intertwining them and producing attributed identities that do not always correspond to the unique experience and identification of each person. Butler, in fact, identifies gender as an instrument for naturalizing sex, making use of discourse to produce the distinction between sexual bodies; making room for the attempt to rationalize, in a social context, allegedly natural relations of power, shaping institutional action and, simultaneously, other individual and collective practices and discourses [7].

In this text, the term trans is adopted in order to emphasize 'the history of the shift from a paradigm of pathology and medical appropriation on gender variability to a new approach that recognizes, and to a large extent through the hands of trans activism, the right of people to designate themselves' [5].

Instead, what we see most of the time is a process in which people identify, define and reframe, plus, attribute a resignification of trans and, after this process, allow themselves to enter into interaction with trans people.

2.3 New perspectives from social relationships with trans people

The Universal Declaration of Human Rights resulted from one of the most serious and heinous ways of selecting people and determining their extermination: the holocaust. Following World War II, in 1948, humanity explicitly states equality through that declaration. As further developed in another text by the first author [8], 'human rights are inherent rights of all human beings, regardless of the place where they are born, conferring nationality, the place where they live, defining cultural norms and the legal and legal norms to which obedience is owed (tacit or mandatory), of the sex with which one is born, of the religion professed and of any other belonging'. The main and distinctive argument is the principle of universality, emphasizing the common element worldwide: to be a human being.

The human rights framework is the broadest approach analyzing social relationships with trans. It is easier to let stereotypes domain in everyday life. In the same way, prejudices emerge unquestionably in social interactions. It is, also, where discrimination occurs and social exclusion takes place.

Seeing the issue from this perspective and knowing that trans persons have become the subject of increased research activity and everyday conversation [9], it is clear that promoting the rights and protection of trans people is a social concern and, therefore, also a political issue. Although it is not assumed that trans persons are a vulnerable population, it is assumed that they may be placed in a vulnerable situation, as they are confronted with stigmatization and transphobia, being sometimes exploited as a weirdo, and not accepted by others [10]. Heteronormative expectations conflict with the idea that a person could be trans. In youth, specifically, trans can be discriminated against and even victims of violence. Furthermore, their gender identity tends to be disrespected, as they are regarded by 'others' as being in the process of 'becoming' and also for being considered that someone only become fully gendered as adults [11]. Recent research dedicated to homophobic bullying, developed in a public school with young people (participating in several focus groups), suggests the acceptance of those who challenge heteronormative expectations—at least among peers, once the study did not involve teachers or other professionals in the school context [12]. In the adult phase of life, research is also being carried out on the acceptance of the labour market and the integration of trans people in the labour market by companies [13]. In fact, the process of building a trans identity is still to be understood in Portugal.

3. The process of right recognition to gender self-determination in Portugal

Internationally, the World Health Organization (WHO), on June 2018, published the 11th version of the Manual for the Classification of Diseases (ICD), where transgender experiences no longer appear as 'sexual identity disorder' (also referred to as 'transsexualism'). Even so, in the V edition of the Diagnostic and Statistical Manual of Mental Disorders (DSM-V) of the American Psychiatric Association (APA), trans people still appear as suffering from a 'gender dysphoria'. This interpretation, in fact, maintains a sexist perspective, when it uses a diagnosis rooted in gender stereotypes of what it is to be a woman or a man, thereby promoting an environment not inclusive of other gender expressions [5].

A few years earlier, in 2009, the International Network for Trans Depathologization, created an international initiative, called Stop Trans Pathologization, with the aim of removing non-normative gender identities from the categories of mental pathologies and disorders. In addition to this objective, it also aimed to revoke the mandatory medical and psychiatric diagnosis for hormonal and surgical treatments and for changing the name and gender in the civil registry.

The 'ideology of legal protection' [14] not always allows us to admit the inability to make an adequate response to sexism, transphobia or misogyny. What is at stake is more than discrimination against people. It is social rights, whether in the sense of access to their effective enjoyment by all people, or in the sense of their inability to cover all people globally, that is, universally. The plurality of gender identity and the diversity of gender intersectionality force us to re-locate the issue in the analysis of processes and not just in the analysis of the result or the impact generated by the result.

A process is a series of actions or steps taken in order to achieve a particular end, distinct, therefore, from a procedure, which is an established or official way of doing something. The process presupposes a duration, and meanwhile, it allows the external influence of other agents on the political position of an agent. Besides, it also allows the same agent to change its interpretation, to review and even change its opinion and/or to get involved in a more participatory way. Moreover, the same agent can distance himself from the debate—either because you lose interest or because you feel that your investment has an unsatisfactory return.

The biomedical model has imposed itself in the social field, expanding its space to areas of behavior previously seen as moral problems or as natural phenomena in the course of life [15]. Despite this, bio-politics, in the case of the regulation of the right to gender self-determination, in Portugal, did not succeed. The legislative framework seems to have favored the opening of space for debate, calling for different positions, including the claim of rights by activist groups inspired by feminism.

In Portugal, the process of building the right to gender self-determination began with a legal-legal perspective, which, in turn, is based on a medical position.

3.1 The Portuguese socio-political context

It is important to situate politically Portugal in the European context, specifically, in the context of Southern Europe. In this context, recent progressive legal transformation coexists with conservative cultural paradigms linked to previous right-wing dictatorships, colonial practices and a powerful Catholic influence, there is a deficit of visibility for lesbian, gay, bisexual, transgender, intersex and queer (LGBTIQ) people throughout history [16].

The individual experiences of trans and non-binary people allow us to retain the importance of the socio-cultural transformation undergone at the micro level, in parallel with the macro-based legal and political advances already studied in the Southern European context [17].

Belgium and Spain show similarities regarding the matters of trans protective rights. In both countries, the regional level has been relevant in introducing trans protective policy. In Belgium, the federal level is responsible for the legislative framework regarding gender recognition. The regional government of Flanders has developed additional extensive policies in order to enhance the well-being, care and equal rights of trans individuals. Similarly, in Spain, a growing number of regions are developing nowadays both trans specific and LGTB antidiscrimination policies, filling the gap that exists at the central state level. In addition, when looking at Trans Rights Europe Map and Index 2017 of Transgender Europe, we see that both countries have developed protective trans legislation at about the same speed [18].

In both Belgium and Spain, additional medical pathways and legal requirements for trans care are demanded, as well as in Portugal.

In turn, the European Parliament in its 2016 Resolution on the application of Council Directive 2000/78/EC of 27 November 2000, establishing a general framework for equal treatment in employment and occupation (called the Employment Equality Directive), called on the Member States and the Commission to combat all forms of multiple discriminations and to ensure application of the principle of non-discrimination and equal treatment in the labour market and in access to employment, increasing monitoring of the intersectionality between gender and other grounds in cases of discrimination and in practices.

The principle of equal treatment, expressed in Article 2 of the Treaty on the European Union and Article 21 of the Charter of Fundamental Rights of the European Union, is a fundamental value of the European Union. The Employment Equality Directive 2000/78/EC forbids discrimination based on sexual orientation only in the context of employment, occupation and training. However, most Member States have extended protection based on sexual orientation, and in some cases, gender identity, to cover some or all fields to which the Race Equality Directive (2000/43/EC) applies. These fields include social security and healthcare, education and access to and supply of goods and services, including housing.

EU law also prohibits sex discrimination in employment and access to goods and services (the Gender Equality Directive (Recast) 2006/54/ EC and the Goods and Services Directive 2004/113/ EC), partly covering trans people.

3.2 Portuguese socio-cultural context

Portugal went through several structural changes that led to the end of a dictatorship, lasting about 50 years. Thus, visibility and space for some themes that were already part of the agenda of other EU Member States were only achieved in Portugal at the end of the first decade of the twenty-first century [19].

It was during this period that the scientific literature began to draw attention to the discrimination and stigmatization of trans people, especially when the gender expression of some trans individuals did not follow traditional gender norms [20–23].

The various social actors place certain identities in a collective social imaginary, composed of social representations, in which trans people are pathologized through biomedical narratives, as they do not integrate the expectations of a binary model in which the genitalia, for a long time, was considered a predictor infallible of each person's gender identity [24].

In Portugal, one of the turning points was the decriminalization of homosexuality in the Penal Code in 1982. Progressively, gender plurality was accepted by society, although initially closely linked to differences between men and women [1]. The first time that the theme of the needs of trans people was on the agenda was through the creation of health responses, linked to surgical intervention aimed at the reassignment of sex. Regulation, once again, marked the process; this time not from a legal perspective, but linked to the ethics of the medical professional practice.

In 1995, the medical profession's regulatory body revoked the prohibition of sex reassignment surgeries in the Code of Ethics, which until then was considered an unethical and illegal practice [25]. The resolution approved on 19 May 1995, by the National Executive Council of the Medical profession's regulatory body, states in article 55, paragraph 1, that 'Surgery for sex reassignment in morphologically normal people is prohibited, except in clinical cases properly diagnosed as transsexualism or like dysphoria'. Following the last authors mentioned, the repeal of the ban on sex reassignment surgeries did not result from pressure exerted by LGBTI activists. In the mid-1990s of the twentieth century in Portugal, collective activist actions were still recent and dispersed. It was only from 2000 onwards that activism formally took over social and legal struggles.

In the process we describe here, this is another turning point, considering that the most organized and most prominent activisms were those on gay and lesbian issues, compared with issues related to bisexuality or specific themes of trans people and women intersex people. Despite the acronym identifying diversity, in reality, only the rights, expectations, needs and the political agenda of gays asserted themselves in Portugal. Even lesbian claims were and continue to be much more dispersed, discrete and with little influence on the political agenda.

It is interesting to know that in Portugal, the trans movement matured and consolidated only after the Gisberta Salce Júnior case, a trans woman victim of homicide, carried out by a group of teenagers, in the city of Porto in 2006 [26]. The attention given by *media* has catapulted a hidden reality marked by social vulnerabilities, which trans person can be targeted, in a way, exposing the fallacies of the Portuguese legal system. Following the social pressure exerted by LGBTI organizations, the small group of organizations specializing in trans issues has become more visible.

Following these events, in 2007, sexual orientation was included in the Penal Code as an aggravating factor in cases of hate crimes. Although this legal advance did not integrate gender identity issues, it represented an achievement for the social movement and reinforced a collective attitude of intolerance towards forms of violence against LGBTI citizens.

In fact, until 2011, the Portuguese legal framework did not contemplate the legal recognition of gender identity. Sex, a natural and birth attribute, continued to be legally considered as an objective, unambiguous factor. In practical terms, that is, in everyday life, a trans citizen had to sue the State to change his name and mention of sex in his civil identification. Only after the bodily transformations could the case lead to the recognition of that person's gender identity [27].

The law that regulated the procedure for changing the sex and changing the name in the civil registry (Law n.° 7/2011, of 15 March), known as the gender identity law, was approved by the Parliament, celebrated by activists and identified by *media* as one of the most progressive laws in the world, for allowing gender to be changed in the personal documentation of each citizen regardless of bodily changes. Corroborating this fact, a report published by Action for Identity in 2015 also states that this was the first law in the world to comply with all Yogyakarta principles, protecting citizens from the obligation to undergo bodily modifications, hormonal treatments or sterilization, different than it was before.

However, from 2015 and 2016, trans and intersex activists began to question aspects they considered obsolete in the law. One of the heavily criticized aspects was the power attributed to medical diagnosis. Although bodily changes due to the use of hormones or surgical procedures are not an aspect taken into account by the Civil Registry in cases of gender recognition, the 2011 law considers a diagnosis to be necessary, carried out by a multidisciplinary team specialized in clinical and surgical sexology, signed by at least one physician and one psychologist, attesting to a gender identity dysphoria, also commonly referred to as transsexuality. Adding to the critique of the pathologized character, activists also point out a need to reduce the bureaucratic burden of this administrative procedure; gender self-determination from 16 years of age onwards; gender recognition for citizens from other countries living in Portugal; the end of any gender-based categories in identification forms and documents; access to other possibilities for gender neutral names; and the prohibition of medical intervention in new-born or intersex child without their consent.

This was the agenda of trans and intersex activists. The bills discussed in parliament included some of these demands, with greater boldness for change in the bills of parties located in the left wing of the Portuguese political party spectrum.

In March 2017, the government presented a final, more consensual version. In this version, changes were made in relation to themes in the health, legal and education areas. Specifically, the biomedical report is no longer mandatory and allows an individual (trans or intersex) aged 16 or over to choose their gender identity. In addition, younger children will be able to choose the name they want to be treated with in schools, regardless of the name on official documents. That is identified as your social name, different from your civil name, which appears in your documentation.

The two bills and the proposed law presented by the government were discussed in the first months of 2018, and the law was approved in April. This process was very intense, as shown in the text below, when we present the results of the study carried out with the main protagonists who participated in the process.

It is now important to bear in mind that in this process, the right to self-determination of gender identity seeks to change pathologized representations towards trans people. Thus, it also breaks with the idea of the existence of a binary gender system, recognizing the right to a plurality of expressions of masculinity and femininity [4, 7].

This very peculiar advance in Portuguese society, which tends to be conservative, was quite important to raise gender issues in the field of human rights. In the Portuguese constitutional system, which is semi-presidential, bills are sent to the president of the republic, who approves or vetoes them. It was precisely in the effective fulfillment of this requirement that, in Portugal, everything seemed to go backwards. Portuguese society in general, activists, social scientists, even a part of the doctors and a part of the deputies in parliament were disappointed.

Decree-Law n. ° 203/XIII, which defined the following: 'Right to self-determination of gender identity and gender expression and to the protection of each person's sexual characteristics', was vetoed (lead) by the President of the Republic in June 2018. The main argument was the prediction of access to self-determination for young people between 16 and 18 years old, without medical supervision. Self-determination turns out to be a critical point. In addition to this, the fact that the doctors did not lead the process was also revealed as a critical point.

The diploma has then returned to parliament. At its plenary meeting on 12 July 2018, the proposed law was approved, providing for the possibility for people aged between 16 and 18 years old to proceed with their process of changing their name and mentioning sex, since accompanied by their legal representatives, and with a medical report attesting to their decision-making capacity and informed will.

Public policies are the result of a negotiation process, with advances and concessions. And, once again, this is demonstrated in the process described here. In addition to this aspect, often referred to in the literature, public policies are always framed by a context. This context, which is external to the political decision process, but which imposes itself on the process, is part of a conservative tradition, a guaranteed way of legislating and an interpretation of the family as determinant, moving away from a perspective of the subject's autonomy. The subject, although he is the holder of rights, enjoys his rights as a member of a family unit. The welfare state has a strong familial bent in Portugal.

The diploma was promulgated (approved) on 31 July 2018, after being modified and resubmitted to the President of the Republic. On 7 August 2018, is published the Law n. ° 38/2018, which defines and regulates the 'Right to self-determination of gender identity and gender expression and to the protection of the sexual characteristics of each person'.

In 2018, Portugal approved a remarkable gender identity law that respects self-determination, because of the concerted work between political actors, academics and activists. The questions that deserved our attention and led us to develop an empirical study were the following: How did social actors interact with each other? What reciprocal influences have occurred?

This text aims to record and analyze the process of formulating the law that established the right to self-determination of gender identity and gender expression and to the protection of each person's sexual characteristics. The achievement of this objective was sought through a qualitative study, using interviews carried out with leaders of the parliamentary groups of political parties represented in Parliament; to activists defending the rights of LGBT people; and to researchers who study the subject scientifically. We have carried out 14 in-depth interviews. The interviews allowed us to identify the reciprocal influence between these social agents and characterize the modes of political pressure most used in the legislative process.

4. The study of public policies advances on trans rights in Portugal

This chapter describes the process of recognizing people's rights through legislative action. In this way, it assumes a critical trans politics perspective instead of a critical approach to resistance. That is, a trans politics demands more than legal recognition and inclusion, seeking to transform current logics of state and social equality. A critical approach does not recognize as useful national stories about social change that actually continues to operate. Besides, a critical approach assumes that public policies and laws are mechanisms used by those with (more) power in society to maintain conditions of suffering and disparity for some—the disempowered ones. Instead, a critical tans politics recognizes legal change in the form of rights as a way of deep transformation [28].

As we said before, the focus of the study and this text is the analysis of the process and not the result or impact of the law. Nor is the focus on analyzing the content of the law. In view of this objective, we explain in more detail the policy analysis process.

4.1 Policy analysis

This text deals with the process of producing a policy (policy process) that refers to the set of methods, strategies and techniques employed in the political resolution of a problem and not the content of that policy (policy content), that is, the essence of matter dealt with [29] —which is analyzed elsewhere.

The analysis of the political process is carried out from the definition of the political agenda in Portugal, including the theme of gender equality in a comprehensive way, to include in the debate the right to gender self-determination.

The agenda is a set of themes that, at a given moment, are perceived by certain political actors as deserving of the State's attention, most of the time in order to correct a situation. In a pragmatic sense, the agenda is a tool that allows organizing problems, favoring an effort to understand their causes and defining possible solutions [30, 31]. The definition of the agenda establishes an order of priorities between themes that do not always follow clear criteria known to others.

The systemic agenda includes issues that gather consensus among the political community as problems that must be resolved, and whose resolution may depend on the Governments. Political decision-makers transfer a part of these issues to the institutional agenda, through pressure, generated by the aggravation of problems or carried out by activists [30]. This internal pressure sometimes coincides with external pressures, which, in the case of Portugal, assume greater importance when they come from the EU and when they result from commitments made by the State [32]. Furthermore, in the virtual space, influence is also exerted on political agendas, which can, in a negative sense, generate some entropy in the collective perceptions that form around a social problem [33].

The political process model, inspired by the contributions of Easton [34], moves away from perspectives that consider the needs, the impulses for social policies. Impulses are factors external to a political system that influence the process of producing social policies, such as public opinion and pressure groups. These present demands or requirements, the demands and keep them continuously in their action. At the same time, they gather support, which assumes different expressions of political support.

The most recent proposal, by Jenkins [29], takes this as a starting point, but it is more useful because it allows integrating the competition between groups and key actors, in a dynamic sense based on a systemic perspective. Thus, the various proposals of a diversity of social actors are considered, in addition to the proposal initially presented [35].

Policy decisions are decisions authorized by political authorities and constitute the pressure for government action that arises both within and outside the political system.

One of the main tools used by interest groups to disseminate their beliefs and views about social reality, whether supported or not by scientific arguments, is the creation of narratives [36, 37].

Narratives are attempts to bring order to a set of complex information. Especially when it comes to information that raises uncertainties, narratives reduce complexity through the creation of stories or scenarios, which can neutralize complex phenomena [2]. One of the main effects that narratives produce on social policies is the reduction of room for negotiation, by conditioning the possibility of new approaches to the problem and by prescribing a set of solutions that tend to be rudimentary [37]. Despite recognizing these biases, the narratives do in fact influence the development of policy-making. They continue to be used because they are instrumental and intrinsic to institutional structures [38]. Therefore, we chose to use the Narrative Policy Framework [39] since it centrally locates the role of policy narratives in the policy process.

4.2 Methodological options in the study of public policies advances on trans rights in Portugal

The Linear Model assumes that policy-makers approach the issues rationally. If we followed a linear model, the flaws would be blamed on a lack of political will, poor management or shortage of resources [37]. In this study, we opted for an analysis of the policy process, as influenced by a range of interest groups that exert power and authority over policy-making. This option makes it clear that we assume a pluralist model that presents policy as primarily reflecting the interests of groups within society.

For the study, we chose as protagonists those most evidently connected and interested in the political process: deputies in parliament; activists, who act as political pressure groups; and the agents who study and, at the same time, define and offer to the other concepts, contribute to marking the barriers to the discussion and to identifying the lines of debate, in a rational and rigorous way. Those names legitimize the debate in the field of science, while the first ones carry out the debate on the political stage of the parliament.

Media were not included in this study, although their power to reinforce and construct alternative narratives is recognized.

The interview was chosen as a data collection technique as it allows the interviewees to elaborate their reasoning only with the orientation of the interviewer (the same in the 14 interviews carried out). The interviews were carried out after the invitation and signing of the informed consent form by each of the interviewees. All interviews were in person and carried out according to the same script and by the same interviewer. The shortest interview lasted about 30 minutes and the longest, about 90 minutes. The transcript, which constituted the corpus of analysis, was subjected to theoretically thematic analysis.

4.3 Main results

This section presents the results of the empirical study, involving different social actors (parliamentary groups, activists and researchers), who were interviewed, individually and separately. One of the objectives is to understand the reciprocal influence between them, despite operating in different stages: the leaders of the parliamentary groups are linked to the *stictu sensu* political process, with the parliament having legislative powers; activists play a fundamental role in a mixed political system and in a democratic regime in which social movements and organized activism can influence the political and legislative process; and researchers produce knowledge about the object of the law and its process as well, analyzing it from a scientific perspective, which is not to be confused with politics or the activist.

All the people interviewed reveal great knowledge and familiarity with the Law, resulting from their involvement with the political process, as deputies or researchers and/or activists heard in parliamentary hearings. In some cases, the people interviewed revealed more than one form of involvement, for example, some deputies simultaneously presented themselves as citizens concerned with the social rights of the trans, and others were simultaneously deputies and activists and/or also experts in area of gender studies.

Five of the 14 interviewees support the designation of trans person as a doctrinal reference used by activists in the trans community, and that they recognize themselves as trans people, coming closer to the conceptual logic of the transgender person, which emphasizes the individual construction of the identity, blurring the experiences of gender as strictly related to the sphere of biology most perceived as a central element in the concept of transsexuality and in pathologize trans people.

It is interesting to point out the opportunity created for social actors to reflect and increase their specific knowledge regarding a proposed law. For example, in one of the interviews it is stated that, 'Regarding the conception I have, it was always a conception that I didn't even question, I didn't know that to say trans instead of saying transgender or transsexual was a political statement'.

Other interviewees look for security in the construction of their political position in international bodies and mechanisms, saying: 'I particularly anchored myself in these guidelines, some of them with the participation of WHO, as you know, WHO on this issue of change It took a long time, but finally it removed issues related to gender change and gender identity from the category of disease'.

The interviewees create, on their own, an association between the conceptual identification and the ideology and political belonging to the party. As one respondent mentioned: 'In political terms, I think there is a tendency for right-wing parties to anchor themselves more to the concept of transsexuality and left-wing parties to the concept of transgender'.

The biomedical model, in turn, emerges as being instrumentalized by conservative political forces. The existence of conceptual tensions that separate ideological-party wings. Specifically, in the narrative of three interviewees, ideological cleavages are an influencing factor on the definition and conceptual references of sex, gender and even on the integration of self-determination for people under 18 years of age.

In this association spontaneously made by the interviewees, one of them refers to the capacity of empathic understanding of certain deputies, from parties more to the right, who internally did not see themselves in the party's position. In an expressive way, an interviewed deputy states that: 'there are positions already taken and it is not exactly scientific knowledge and what we are told changes positions, this was noted in this case'.

Another respondent admits that there are overlapping political commitments, namely the need to maintain the electorate, for example, by constraining a party position aligned with a human rights framework. Thus, there are only three interviewees who place the social rights of trans people within the framework of human rights, adopting it as their reference.

From the interviewees' point of view, among the main triggers for public and political discussion is political intention or will. The government's programme has been an essential factor, because it contained the intention to legislate on this topic—specifically in the chapter entitled 'Building a more equal society', in which it is explained that the intention is to 'improve the regime of gender identity, namely in the which concerns the need to provide for the civil recognition of intersex people and to improve the legislative framework for transsexual and transgender people' [40].

Another trigger that drives the legislative process itself is activist work and scientific investigation. These emerge in the interviewees' speeches as the main tools for integrating the theme in the public space of debate and in the political agenda. The penetration into the institutional agenda of the right to gender self-determination, gender expression and protection of sexual characteristics may have been the culmination of a path guided mainly by social actors outside the political arena, in the strictest sense, such as activists and researchers.

Immediately afterwards, the individual perception of the availability of political decision-makers to incorporate scientific contributions and associations in the decision-making process emerges in their speeches. The majority of interviewees, 11 out of 14, believe that scientific contributions and/or those arising from the pressure of movements or associative processes may have calibrated the discussion in light of the initial opposition to the idea of gender self-determination by some political forces.

Nevertheless, the remaining respondents believe that the valuation exists, but up to a point. One of the interviewees mentions that scientific contributions should be even more valued in the decision-making process of some parliamentary groups, which sometimes have positions previously taken even before scientific considerations.

5. Final remarks

The study of policy process on advances on rights of trans persons in Portugal confirms that when rights are guaranteed through public policy, the probability of becoming 'de facto' rights rather than just 'de jure' rights is greatly increased.

The interviews reveal that when reflecting on gender identity in the political sphere, it is not always clear that gender is also a discursive medium that situates certain identities in a collective social imaginary, composed of social representations, in which trans people have been pathologized by the biomedical model, for not integrating the expectations of a binary model in which the genitalia, for a long time, was considered an infallible predictor of gender identity.

The study also revealed that the interaction between activists and some political decision makers is productive, namely in the assimilation of some concepts and in the appropriation of reflexive logics. This interaction is also seen as productive because it is instrumental, improving parliamentary contributions and interactions with the *media*. Even so, some policy-makers are selective about what they listen to and what they integrate into their political agendas, especially concerning structural issues.

Lastly, it emphasizes the importance of analyzing the political process from theoretical models that invite us to observe each of the interveners and the interaction between them, admitting also that the interpretation of a theme as a problem influences the outcome of this political process.

Acknowledgments

This work was funded by national funds through FCT - Fundação para a Ciência e Tecnologia, I.P., under project UIDP/04304/2020.

Author details

Dalia Costa[1] and Miguel Miranda[2]*

1 Interdisciplinary Centre for Gender Studies, Research Centers of the Institute of Social and Political Sciences, University of Lisbon (ISCSP-ULisboa), Lisbon, Portugal

2 Higher Institute of Social and Political Sciences (ISCSP) of University of Lisbon, Lisbon, Portugal

*Address all correspondence to: miguelmiranda001@gmail.com

References

[1] Amâncio L. O género no discurso das Ciências Sociais. Análise Social. 2003;**168**:687-714

[2] Dias I. Matrizes Teóricas da Violência de Género. In: Neves S, Costa D, editors. Violências de Género. Lisboa: ISCSP; 2017. pp. 23-44

[3] Bourdieu P. La Domination Masculine. France: Éditions du Seuil; 1998

[4] Connell R. Gênero. Uma Perspectiva Global. Brasil: nVersos; 2015

[5] Rodrigues L, Carneiro N, Nogueira C. Violência Transfóbica: Aproximações Críticas e Horizontes de Resistência. In: Neves S, Costa D, editors. Violência de Género. Lisboa: ISCSP; 2017. pp. 261-282

[6] Griffin G. A Dictionary of Gender Studies. OUP Oxford: Oxford Quick Reference Online; 2017

[7] Butler J. Problemas de Género. Lisboa: Orfeu Negro; 2017

[8] Costa D. Violência de Género, Igualdade e Direitos Humanos. In: Neves S, Costa D, editors. Violências de Género. Lisboa: Edições ISCSP; 2017. pp. 261-282

[9] Turner L, Whittle S, Combs R. Transphobic Hate Crime in the European Union. London: Press for Change; 2009

[10] Hines S, Santos A. Trans* policy, politics and research: The UK and Portugal. Critical Social Policy. 2018;**38**(1):35-56. DOI: ttps://doi.org/10.1177/0261018317732880

[11] Olson-Kennedy J, Cohen-Kettenis P, Kreukels B, Meyer-Bahlburg H, Garofalo R, Meyer M, et al. Research priorities for gender nonconforming/transgender youth: Gender identity development and biopsychosocial outcomes. Current Opinion in Endocrinology, Diabetes, and Obesity. 2016;**23**(2):172-179. DOI: 10.1097/MED.0000000000000236

[12] Costa D, Santos L. Students' perspectives on bullying: Peer standards setting process unveiled in focus groups. British Educational Research Journal. 2022 (submitted)

[13] Costa D, Baptista J. Be trans and worker: Processes in accessing the labor market. Gender & Society. 2022 (submitted)

[14] Bumiller K. In an Abusive State: How Neoliberalism Appropriated the Feminist Movement against Sexual Violence. Durham, North Carolina, USA: Duke University Press; 2008

[15] Ferreira da Silva L. Saúde comunitária: riscos e potencialidades da participação. Alicerces. Lisboa: Edições Colibri, Instituto Politécnico de Lisboa; 2010:65-78. Retrieved from: https://www.ipl.pt/sites/default/files/alicerces_3.pdf

[16] Santos A. Strategic identity and self-determination within the LGBTQI+ framework. Posts by Discover Society. 2020:77. Retrieved from: https://archive.discoversociety.org/2020/02/05/strategic-identity-and-self-determination-within-the-lgbtqi-framework/

[17] Cascais F. Indisciplinar a Teoria. Estudos Gays, Lésbicos e Queer. Lisboa: Fenda; 2004

[18] see http://tgeu.org/trans-rights-map-2017/)

[19] Torres A, Costa D, Sant'Ana H, Coelho B. Sexual Harrassment and Bullying in the Workplace in Portugal. Lisboa: CITE; 2016

[20] Drydakis N. Trans People, Well-Being, and Labor Market Outcomes. IZA World of Labor, September, article number 386. Germany: IZA; 2017. pp. 1-9. DOI: 10.15185/izawol. Retrieved from: https://www.econstor.eu/handle/10419/171194

[21] Leppel J. The labor force status of transgender men and women. International Journal of Transgenderism. 2017;**17**(3-4):155-164

[22] Monro S, Van Der Ros J. Trans and gender variant citizenship and the state in Norway. Critical Social Policy. 2017;**38**:1-22. DOI: 10.1177026101831 7733084

[23] Missé M. Transsexualidades: Outras Miradas Posibles. 2° ed. Barcelona, Madrid: Egales Editorial; 2014

[24] Saleiro S. Trans Géneros: Uma Abordagem Sociológica da Diversidade de Género PhD dissertation. Lisbon: ISCTE-IUL; 2013

[25] Hines S, Santos A. Trans* policy, politics and research: The UK and Portugal. Critical Social Policy. 2018;**38**(1):35-56. DOI: 10.1177/0261018317732880

[26] Rodrigues C. Gisberta, 10 anos depois: a diva transexual que acabou no fundo do poço. Observador. 2016. Retrieved from https://observador.pt/especiais/gisberta-10-anos-diva-homofobia-atirou-fundo-do-poco/

[27] Pinto N. Experiencing and Representing Transsexuality: Devolopment Trajectories of, and Social Representations on, Transsexual People. ISCTE: Lisboa; 2014

[28] Spade D. Introduction: Rights, movements, and critical trans politics. In: Normal Life: Administrative Violence, Critical Trans Politics, and the Limits of Law. New York: Duke University Press; 2015. DOI: 10.1515/9780822374794-002

[29] Jenkins W. Policy analysis: Models and approaches. In: Hill M, editor. The Policy Process: A Reader. 2nd ed. Hertfordshire: Prentice Hall; 1997. pp. 30-38

[30] Buck S. Understanding Environmental Administration and Law. Washington DC: Island Press; 1996

[31] Turner B. The Cambridge Dictionary of Sociology. United States of America: Cambridge University Press; 2006

[32] Börzel T. How the European Union Interacts with its Member States. Reihe Politikwissenschaft - Political Science Series 93. Wien: Institut für Höhere Studien (IHS) - Vienna: Institute for Advanced Studies; 2003. Retrieved from: https://www.ihs.ac.at/publications/pol/pw_93.pdf

[33] Aelst P, Thesen G, Walgrave S, Vliegenthart R. Mediatization and political agenda-setting: Changing issue priorities? In: Esser F, Strömbäck J, editors. Mediatization of Politics: Understanding the Transformation of Western Democracies. London: Palgrave Macmillan; 2014. pp. 200-220

[34] Hill M. The Policy Process in the Modern State. 3rd ed. Hertfordshire: Prentice Hall; 1997

[35] Hilgartner J, Bosk C. The rise and fall of social problems: A public arenas model. American Journal of Sociology. 1988;**40**:53-78

[36] Elizabeth A, McBeth M, Arnell R, Hathaway P. Conduit or contributor?

The role of Media in Policy Change Theory. Policy Sciences. 2008;**41**(2):115-138

[37] Sutton R. The Policy Process: An Overview. Working Paper 118. London SW1E 5DP. ISBN: 0 85003 417 5: Overseas Development Institute. Portland House Stag Place; 1999

[38] Leach M, Mearns R. The Lie of the Land: Challenging Received Wisdom on the African Environment. Oxford: James Currey; 1996

[39] Jones M, McBeth M. A narrative policy framework: Clear enough to Be wrong? The Policy Studies Journal. 2010;**38**(2):329-353. Available at: http://works.bepress.com/mjones/3

[40] Program of the XXI Constitutional Government. 2015. Retrieved from: https://www.portugal.gov.pt/ficheiros-geral/programa-do-governo-pdf.aspx

Chapter 4

Perspective Chapter: Transitioning to Transgender – How Can We Help?

Phaedra E. Cress

Abstract

Change is not easy in a professional environment and it is even more challenging in our personal lives. In this chapter, I explore how we can all become champions of the transgender population. My interest in the transgender population started 3 years ago when my child came out as transgender. My daughter is now a son and I have become an ally of the LGBTQ+ community. I have learned to embrace the journey and am continuously learning how I can support and elevate the transgender community in myriad ways. I share the experiences that have shaped my life recently with the hope it might help others, particularly parents of transgender children, understand one simple idea: "you are not alone".

Keywords: transgender, LGBTQ+, diversity, inclusion, microaggression, survivor, pronouns, anxiety, depression

1. Introduction

> "You deserve the best, the very best, because you are one of the few people in this lousy world who are honest to themselves, and that is the only thing that really counts."
>
> —Frida Kahlo

You are not alone. That phrase resonates with me as the parent of a transgender son. We live in a new era that welcomes changes in gender, identity, and sexual orientation. Unlike past generations who chastised and criminalized those who were different, we now have an established vernacular that continues to evolve toward inclusivity and equality. Among this community is the transgender population comprised of trans men who were assigned as females at birth and trans women who were assigned as men at birth. The transgender population deserves to not only be understood but embraced for their important contributions and authenticity. They deserve our attention and the empathy and sympathy of the personal and professional communities in which they work [1]. They deserve to be their authentic selves without fear of microaggressions and discrimination.

2. Discussion

In this chapter, I explore the following key points to help put these concepts into perspective; (1) How can everyone champion the transgender population and understand their unique population? (2) How should the transgender be cared for, communicated with, and psychologically related to as is done so naturally for cisgender men and women? (3) What society's obligation in this context and what resources exist? The author also discusses her personal experiences relative to her transgender son and their journey together with the hopes it will guide those on a similar path now or in the future.

My impressions and personal interest in the transgender population began 3 years ago when my child expressed that his contrary to his biological gender, he believed his true gender was male. To illuminate my journey, I offer readers a view into the experiences that have shaped my life in the years since I became mother to a transgender son with the hopes that it might help others understand one simple idea: you are not alone.

There are myriad resources for parents of transgender children and while every transgender person may be on their own path to discovery and personal enlightenment, we cannot discount the ripple effect of the parents, families, friends, and by extension all those with whom a transgender person interacts.

There is a strong connection between the psychological, emotional, and physical feelings of dysphoria and confusion, especially when trans men and women begin their transition. There is beauty in a name especially when chosen as the first step of a brand-new journey in discovering oneself. Imagine the satisfaction that must come with re-branding oneself in a movement toward transitioning to a new gender. What's in a name? Simply put: everything. Hearing your chosen name used for the very first time by those around you is one of the first steps toward social acceptance and self-awareness. My son chose to use his initials (A. J.) as an interim name while he selected Drew as his formal new name. Retraining myself after 13 years to call my child by these new names wasn't easy but it was critically important, so he understood immediately that I was by his side, his lifelong champion, and that my love was unconditional. Surprisingly, it was my younger son who was faster at adapting and remember to use the new name, an unexpected resilience that helped our family in so many ways.

Another valuable lesson learned was the huge impact of using preferred pronouns to help the transgender immediately begin to feel more like themselves and more accepted by their family, friends, and community. I've known many parents of trans men and women who've expressed their own discomfort and inability to bring themselves to make this change or to call their child by their new name. I cannot judge them any more than I'd want them to judge me. However, it quickly became apparent to me that in my situation, the significance of names and pronouns and the power they held for my child could not be overstated. In this sense, I realized I had to quickly adopt both as the first steps in his transition.

Consider how long some transgender people wait to share their true feelings and how by accommodating this request you can illustrate your support for them. I have known transgender men and women who were married for decades and then finally shared their true gender with their spouse. Some were accepted and are living harmoniously and for others it destroyed their relationship. Many trans men use the pronouns he/him and many trans women use the pronouns she/her. Some who identify as nonbinary may prefer they/their pronouns. Using the appropriate and preferred pronouns shows respect and care for those with whom you interact and is one important way to champion the transgender community [2]. Making gender assumptions based on appearance could send a harmful message or be interpreted as offensive. Leadership by example, set by someone who uses pronouns, may be the paradigm to make your coworkers feel more connected, inspired, or empowered to bring their "true self" to work every day and contribute in a more passionate and meaningful way. Leaders and peers should all be encouraged to express their authenticity freely and without fear of judgement. It may be a very small gesture for the cisgender but can have a life-changing effect for the transgender. Using the incorrect pronouns, whether intentionally or not, is known as "misgendering." This show of disrespect can trigger dysphoria and embarrassment for some individuals because it forces them to have painful conversations and reveal identity information about themselves they may not be comfortable sharing publicly. The sharing of preferred pronouns in business, among both cisgender and the transgender community, has become more popular. But are all the ramifications positive? I include my personal pronouns in the signature of every email I send plus a descriptive informational link as: Pronouns: She/Her/Hers Why pronouns? As the mother of a transgender, I feel ownership about the need to help educate others about the importance of pronouns, which I hope will lead to broader understanding, acceptance, and usage. International Pronouns Day began in 2019 on the third Wednesday in October as an effort to create a more inclusive environment for everyone to "make respecting, sharing, and educating about personal pronouns commonplace" [3]. I appreciated this quote from the International Pronouns Day website:

"Trans and nonbinary people often have to share their pronouns to be identified correctly. As a cisgender person, sharing pronouns costs nothing and naturalizes this process."

A more generalized set of personal pronouns that evolved from the transgender community and are becoming more widely adopted as gender-neutral are: xe/xir/xem/xeir and ze/zir/zirs [4]. Using the correct pronouns may be particularly challenging in a work environment but as the movement toward better diversity and inclusivity continues to evolve, the conversation has become more important than ever. A McKinsey and Company survey shows that 39% of potential job candidates turned down an offer because they perceived the organization to lack inclusivity in their workplace and 84% of respondents experienced microaggressions in the workplace, everyday slights or biases against them, such as negative remarks about their identity or how they dress, being asked to speak for or represent "people like them" or to correct assumptions of colleagues about their personal lives. Thirty-nine percent of LGBTQ+ respondents were uncomfortable sharing their LGBTQ+ identity with colleagues, or "coming out" to them and 37% responded the interactions were slightly or very uncomfortable [5]. My main motivation is to empower my child and contribute to a world where his path is easier if even in some small way, so he and others are spared unnecessary bias and judgement.

In addition to selecting a new name and surrounding oneself with those willing to help them transition by using their pronouns, for the female to male (FTM) transgender population there is another crucial stage of the transition process: chest binding [6]. Binding affords them another tool in the FTM armamentarium: to look and feel more cisgender. I have witnessed firsthand how binding can help alleviate dysphoria and enable an FTM to present as a cisgender male whose identity pairs more naturally with how they feel authentically. Wearing a compression binder helps flatten the breast and can avoid the embarrassment of looking like a woman or being judged by peers. It is important for parents to monitor their children's use of binders because wearing sizes that are too small in an effort to "look more flat" can make it difficult to breathe, especially when playing sports, in gym class, or on hot and humid days. It's also important to know that trans men do not have to bind for the rest of their lives. Once a decision is made to begin a testosterone regimen, eventually the breast will become smaller and menses will stop, both of which are huge developmental and emotional improvements during a transition. Using kinetic tape is another binding method with which I am less familiar, but it could also be effective if care it taken to avoid sensitive skin irritation. According to WebMD finding the right size binder is crucial because failure to do so can cause overheating and rib bruising or even fracture and it's especially challenging for anyone with asthma, scoliosis, Lupus, or Fibromyalgia [5]. It is also important to monitor those who bind because sleeping with a binder on is not recommended. Like everything, the body needs time to rest and recuperate and more than 8 h of binding can cause longer-term health issues.

Once a transgender person has conquered the beginning stages of their transition and are supported by their family, friends, and co-workers with the use of their new name, preferred pronouns, and they have begun dressing and feeling more like their authentic identity, it may be time to consider puberty blockers or hormone therapy. Puberty blockers will help reduce the growth of breast tissue and block menses and are an accepted and universal first step in the transition process. They are, however, very costly, and sometimes unaffordable. The use of puberty blockers is understood to be reversible—meaning if there was a desire to return to one's biological gender, there would be no adverse long-term effects. The use of hormone therapy offers no guarantee about reversibility, and in fact it is generally understood that using them is *not* reversible and *may* contribute to long-term effects such as an increase/reduction in hair growth, changes to the voice, and more masculinized or feminized body features that result from hormone therapy. The process involves an initial consultation with a pediatrician and referral to an endocrinologist (typically one who specializes in transgender patients). It is also important to seek out a therapist, psychiatrist, or psychologist with transgender experience who can help guide those transitioning during or throughout the process to ensure their mental and emotional wellbeing.

The World Professional Association for Transgender Health (WPATH) and the Endocrine Society created guidelines for doctors to help care for the transgender community and to ensure all decisions are as evidence-based as possible and appropriate for the age and stage of the transition. According to Unger, hormone therapy for trans men is based on treatment of hypogonadal natal men whereas estrogen therapy for trans women is based on the treatment of postmenopausal women. The hormones are most typically administered intramuscularly on a regular basis by needle injection [7]. A study by Korpaisarn et al. applied the 2017 Endocrine Society Clinical Practice Guideline for the Endocrine Treatment of Gender-Dysphoric/Gender-Incongruent Persons and found that within the first 6 months of testosterone treatment, the study participants developed skin oiliness, acne, cessation of menses, increased facial hair, deepening of the voice. After 6 months, they observed an increased muscle mass, body hair [8]. According to Cirrincione and Huang there are 25 million transgender people 15 years or older yet clinical pharmacology for transgender medicine has fallen behind [9]. Grant et al. found that 70% of transgender adults reported taking hormone therapy [10].

Some in the transgender community talk about being survivors because they are faced with the challenge of chronic misgendering in addition to things we take for granted such as using public restrooms (or in the case of school-aged children, locker rooms), public showers at the gym, and swimming in pools and at beaches. I have observed this in my own child, a complete reticence to wear a bathing suit because of his dysphoria. But do they identify as being survivors because of their identity change or are they survivors of their past identity (or "dead name" as many call their birth name)? Budge et al. looked at anxiety and depression in the transgender population and found it was higher than in the general population. They found that symptoms of depression were present 51.4% of transgender women and 48.3% for transgender men and symptoms of anxiety were found in 40.4% of transgender women and 47.5% for transgender men [11].

How else can the world at large help offset the psychological turmoil felt by this population? A new study in the *Journal of Adolescent Health* by Turban et al. [12] looked at the timing of transition, harassment during elementary, middle school, and high school, and mental health outcomes in adults. The study reports on more than 27,000 transgender men and women who transitioned at different times (ages 3–9; ages 10–17; or 18 and older). They found those who transitioned in adulthood (18 or older) experienced higher use of marijuana and lifetime suicide attempts but an equally important factor was having a safe and affirming social environment that avoids harassment between grades K and 12. In an aptly named article by Andrzejewski et al., "Perspectives of Transgender Youth on Parental Support: Qualitative Findings From the Resilience and Transgender Youth Study," [13] the authors looked at the intervention of parental support on outcomes in this population. While there is a general paucity of information and data to address this data point, they interviewed 33 parents of transgender youth, looking at these forms of support: (1) emotional; (2) instrumental; (3) appraisal; (4) informational. While they found a general support for their child's transition, it was more limited than expected, indicating parents could benefit from help and information to help gender-affirming behaviors and transitions.

One of the most dynamic and useful resources I have found is this one: https://pflag.org/. Nine days after my son told me he was transgender I was referred to this group, which meets locally throughout the country. It is a diverse group of transgender boys, girls, men, women and their parents. Prior to COVID, we met monthly and the support, guidance, and knowledge I gained has been invaluable throughout my journey with my son. During some of the most challenging times, the group has provided support and perspective and I often left feeling humbled by the experiences of others and grateful to know they understood what my son and I were going through from personal experience.

3. Conclusions

Whether you are considering a transition or are guiding a loved one through the journey, there are a few simple steps you can take to be a champion and to be a survivor and to help someone navigate their own journey. The easiest first step is to begin using pronouns in the workplace in their email signatures, on video conference calls, and referring to colleagues with their preferred pronouns [14, 15]. This helps support the transgender community and allows the freedom of expression among their cisgender peers [14, 15]. I encourage you to learn all that you can to help the transgender population because it will have exponentially positive ripple effects as we all work toward improvements in diversity and inclusion. I never suspected that I would become a tangential part of the LGBTQ+ community, but now that I am, I feel it is a unique honor to participate in any way I can to help educate, guide, and counsel those around me who need support. Issues of diversity, epidemiology, and mental health are interrelated and must be carefully observed in the transgender population, especially by parents and close associates to ensure their mental and physical stability [16–20]. This population is more prone to mental health issues and suicidal ideation as a result of the social issues and physical dysphoria they face. It is critical that public policy, laws, and social practices be improved to avoid transgender discrimination and marginalization because even plastic surgery procedures such as gender-affirming facial procedures and top surgery are not effective without such reform because mental health issues will persist [21].

Sharing what I've learned and helping those who I can has been one of the most rewarding experiences of my life. Where I initially felt I was not capable of managing all the emotions and challenges and questions, I now impart to others that it will be OK, you can survive. It is critical to remember that gender does not define who your child is; they will always be your child. Being their champion and ultimate supporter will help them become the incredible individual they were meant to be. We all go through the experience at a different pace and there is no right or wrong in this regard. The best advice I can offer is to love your child unconditionally so they will love themselves unconditionally. Everything begins with knowing they are supported, loved, and understood so the lessons they've learned can be taken forward with positivity and creativity to help them evolve into a strong and confident person who knows their value and is proud of themselves. We parents may not have all the answers and may sometimes feel as if we have nothing but questions, but you're now raising a survivor and that means you, too, are a survivor. Good luck, and Godspeed my friends!

Author details

Phaedra E. Cress
Aesthetic Surgery Journal, Garden Grove, USA

*Address all correspondence to: pecress@gmail.com

References

[1] Cress P. We are the champions: Caring for the transgender. Aesthetic Surgery Journal. 2021;**41**(3):388-390. DOI: 10.1093/asj/sjaa353

[2] Spirgel C. It's about basic respect-making pronoun sharing the standard. Includr. 2021. Available from: https://includr.org/practice/its-about-basic-respect-making-pronoun-sharing-the-standard/?gclid=Cj0KCQiA2NaNBhDvARIsAEw55hjEczvE498X82nWBJNL5P0Oz_fu27AarrIVlXXjddUSqezJ8atobHoaApnPEALw_wcB. [Accessed: 02 December 2 2021]

[3] International pronouns day. Available from: https://pronounsday.org/. [Accessed: 12 December 2021]

[4] My pronouns are. Pronouns.page. Available from: https://en.pronouns.page/ze/zir [Accessed: 11 December 2021]

[5] Understanding Organizational Barriers to a More Inclusive Workplace. McKinsey and Company. 2020. Available from: https://www.mckinsey.com/business-functions/people-and-organizational-performance/our-insights/understanding-organizational-barriers-to-a-more-inclusive-workplace [Accessed: 09 December 2021]

[6] Brennan D. What is chest binding? WebMD. April 9, 2021. Available from: https://www.webmd.com/a-to-z-guides/what-is-chest-binding#:~:text=Chest%20binding%20has%20become%20a,female%2Dto%2Dmale%20transition. [Accessed: 05 December 2021]

[7] Unger CA. Hormone therapy for transgender patients. Translational Andrology and Urology. 2016;**5**(6):877-884. DOI: 10.21037/tau.2016.09.04

[8] Korpaisarn S et al. Effects of testosterone treatment on transgender males: A single-institution study. SAGE Open Medicine. 2021;**9**:1-9. DOI: 10.1177/20503121211051546

[9] Cirrincione LR, Huang KH. Sex and gender differences in clinical pharmacology: Implications for transgender medicine. Clinical Pharmacology & Therapeutics. 2021;**110**(4):897-908. DOI: 10.1002/cpt.2234

[10] Grant JM, et al. Injustice at every turn: A report of the national transgender discrimination survey. Available from: https://transequality.org/sites/default/files/docs/resources/NTDS_Report.pdf. [Accessed: 07 December 2021]

[11] Budge S, Adelson JL, Howard KAS. Anxiety and depression in transgender individuals: The roles of transition status, loss, social support, and coping. Journal of Consulting and Clinical Psychology. 2013;**81**(3):545-557. DOI: 10.1037/a0031774

[12] Turban JL et al. Timing of social transition for transgender and gender diverse youth, K-12 harassment, and adult mental health outcomes. Journal of Adolescent Health. 2021;**69**(6):991-998

[13] Andrzejewski J et al. Perspectives of transgender youth on parental support: Qualitative findings from the resilience and transgender youth study. Health Education and Behavior. 2021;**48**(1):74-81

[14] Cress P. The power of personal pronouns to encourage diversity and inclusion. Aesthetic Surgery Journal 2022. DOI: 10.1093/asj/sjac087. [Epub ahead of print]

[15] Goodman M, Adams N, Corneil T, Hashemi L, Kreukels B, Swan J, et al. Mental health and quality of life outcomes of gender-affirming surgery: A systematic literature review. Journal of Gay & Lesbian Mental Health. pp. 1-44. DOI: 10.1080/19359705.2021.2016537

[16] Koehler A, Motmans J, Mulió Alvarez L, Azul D, Badalyan K, Basar K, et al. How the COVID-19 pandemic affects transgender health care—A cross-sectional online survey in 63 upper-middle-income and high-income countries. International Journal of Transgender Health. 2021:1-14

[17] Ghassabian A, Suleri A, Blok E, Franch B, Hillegers MHJ, White T. Adolescent gender diversity: Sociodemographic correlates and mental health outcomes in the general population. Journal of Child Psychology & Psychiatry. 2022;**20**. DOI: 10.1111/jcpp.13588

[18] Stryker SD, Palleria H, Yockey RA, Berdad-Thomas J, Pickle S. Training mental health professionals in gender-affirming care: A survey of experienced clinicians. Transgender Health. 2022;**7**(1):68-77

[19] Rutnin S, Suchonwanit P, Kositkulijorn C, Pomsoong C, Korpaisarn S, Arunakul J, et al. Characterizing dermatological conditions in the transgender population: A cross-sectional study. Transgender Health. 2022;**13**. DOI: 10.1089/trgh.2021.0105 [Epub ahead of print]

[20] Lett E, Everhart A. Considerations for transgender population health research based on US national surveys. Annals of Epidemiology. 2022;**65**:65-71

[21] Swan J, Phillips TM, Sanders T, Mullens AB, Debattista J, Brömdal A. Mental health and quality of life outcomes of gender-affirming surgery: A systematic literature review. Journal of Gay & Lesbian Mental Health. 2022. DOI: 10.1080/19359705.2021.2016537

Chapter 5

Health of Trans People in Paraguay

Carlos Miguel Rios-González

Abstract

Trans care is not taught in conventional medical education programs, and very few doctors have the knowledge and comfort level to do so. A theoretical design study was carried out using the bibliographic review method, which allowed to provide a systematic framework of products in terms of scientific publications and official publications on the health of transgender people. In the Paraguayan context, it is recognized that sex work is the main economic activity of 86% of trans people, which although it is a job that is not punished in Paraguay, but neither is it recognized or regulated by law, although in Paraguay, numerous international instruments for the protection of human rights have been ratified, by which it is obliged to adopt measures to guarantee the sexual and reproductive health of all people and nondiscrimination based on sex, sexual orientation, and gender identity.

Keywords: transgender, health, LGTB+ collective, trans people, Paraguay

1. Introduction

The LGTB+ collective (lesbians, gays, transsexuals, and bisexuals) has acquired in recent years greater recognition of its affective-sexual diversity and with it, greater visibility in society [1]. Although the policies for the representation of this group at the community level have been updated, numerous studies continue to show the discrimination suffered by LGTB individuals, particularly the group of trans people, who are more frequently victimized even through the use of powers in public in each country [2].

Gender identity is one of the determining aspects in a person's life. Likewise, biological sex is a condition that is assigned to us at birth based on primary sexual characteristics, a corporality that will later constitute both a legally and socially binding factor [3]. Both concepts are in interaction in the person and may or may not coincide according to what is culturally established [4].

By trans people, we will understand all those who do not recognize themselves in the sex assigned at birth and build, assume, and identify themselves and others as trans men or women; consequently, it is usual for them to want to change their names, do some medical or surgical intervention, or position themselves from another place of gender different from the normative one according to their sexual assignment [5].

The foregoing is based especially on the fact that their identity constructions go beyond the binary conception of gender, according to which there is a natural relationship and full correspondence between sex and gender [6, 7]. This sustains a system of oppression, under which "everyone" must identify and recognize themselves as they were assigned at birth, and becomes the most legitimized by society, generating as a consequence segregation, discrimination, and violence against anyone who identifies in a different way to those established and that are not normative [1].

The scenario that trans people face, with respect to the development and expression of their experiences and the construction of their gender identities, in Colombian society at the time of receiving medical care, makes it necessary to specify the definitions of the key concepts that make up these processes and that allow us to understand that they are different for each individual [3]. They are constantly nurtured from diverse identity experiences and therefore deserve that the whole of society and health providers respect and recognize their diversity [5].

The transgender population faces a social and historical problem, since the establishment of the so-called "sexual dimorphism" established in the eighteenth century, from which a whole culture arises to name the anatomical variations of the bodies, and the supposed correspondence of this with gender, whether feminine or masculine [1, 6]. All this has been implanted as an ideal for many centuries in people, causing a marginalization of everything that is outside these terms, which can also be expressed as limits.

In the field of health, there is a misunderstanding due to the differences that make up their identities, corporalities, and gender expressions, in the same way that happens in other areas of society, making it necessary for there to be an adequate provision for their needs and particularities. A situation that has given rise to discrimination, artisanal medical practices, apathy toward the health system, among others; hindering the free development of the personality of these people and the right to a life in conditions of dignity and equality [7]. The foregoing has meant that they direct their struggles so that the State and health providers guarantee adequate and continuous care, which has been materialized in different normative instruments at the international and national levels, as explained below.

2. Methodology

A theoretical design study was carried out using the bibliographic review method, which allowed to provide a systematic framework of products in terms of scientific publications and official publications on the health of transgender people.

The units of analysis were scientific articles of primary type, located through seven databases recognized for their scientific rigor. In addition, the official web pages of activist and/or related groups were searched.

The search equation used in the keywords field (KW) was: "Health" AND "Transgender," "Trans" OR "LGBT" AND "Paraguay." These keywords do not necessarily correspond to thesauri, since they were chosen to ensure the widest possible number of articles published on the subject.

The search for documents included the Spanish, English, and Portuguese languages, no time period restriction was applied, and that they had been published and/or carried out in scientific journals and official web pages of activist and/or related groups.

A database of bibliographic records was generated to describe each unit of analysis with the following inductive categories: (a) bibliographic data: author and year of publication; (b) study objective and most important findings; (c) contextual variables: country where the study was conducted; (d) methodological variables: instruments and data collection techniques used. From the analysis of the bibliographic records, the deductive categories emerged: application method, study method, models, and evaluation.

3. Key concepts

Currently, the demand for health care from trans people is more frequent, so it is necessary for the doctor, even if he is not a specialist, to know general aspects regarding terminology, health needs, legal medical treatment, and considerations regarding possible effects of medical treatments to which these patients are subjected in their transition to felt gender identity [8].

To analyze this topic, it is necessary to define the terms: sex, gender, sexual determination, sexual orientation [9].

- Sex is defined according to the biological determinants of the individual; In most cases, newborns are assigned as male or female according to their anatomical sex, which, for the social context, should seek to be consistent with a "masculine" (as a child) or "feminine" gender identity and expression (of girl). In the event that the newborn does not have a defined anatomical sex, the term intersex is used (previously called hermaphrodites) [10].

- Gender refers to the internal personal experience of feeling masculine, feminine, or androgynous, depending on the cultural context (gender identity). The World Health Organization (WHO) defines it as "characteristics of men and women that are based on social factors, while sex refers to characteristics that are biologically determined." If the person identifies with the sex assigned at birth, they are considered a "cisgender" person, if they do not, they are considered "transgender" [9].

The expression of gender that encompasses aspects of behavior in which men and women are different according to culture and historical stage (male or female gender behavior according to cultural patterns). In recent decades, it is more common to see expressions of gender behaviors other than those classically known as masculine or feminine, including people who are androgynous, bigenders, or who do not identify with either of the two genders (non-binary).

- Sexual orientation refers to whom the sexual desire is directed toward, existing people with homo, hetero, bisexual, pansexual, demisexual orientation, none (asexual), etc., depending on where the individual's erotic-affective attraction is directed, which it is not necessarily defined by the sex assigned at birth [9].

In short, we will have individuals with:

- Chromosomal sex XX, XY and its variants.

- Male, female, or intersex genital sex.

- heterosexual, bisexual, asexual, demisexual, or pansexual sexual orientation.

- Sexual appearance determined by the phenotypic aspect and by the expression of masculine, feminine, or androgynous gender identity or expression, depending on the cultural context of the individual [10].

Thus, we can see that sex, gender, and sexual orientation are not synonyms.

Finished	Definition
Gender	Cultural construction that assigns, in the public and private sphere, forms of behavior and roles to women and men based on their sexual differentiation (WHO definition)
Gender identity	Internal feeling of the individual (not visible to others), of being male or female
Gender variants	Individual with gender expression that differs from social expectations related to the assigned gender
Transgender	Gender identity, expression and behavior differs from the gender assigned at birth
Cisgender	Gender identity, expression and behavior concordant with the gender assigned at birth
Non-binary gender	Disagreement with any of the two classic forms of gender (male-female)
Transgender man	Person with female sexual characteristics, identified as female at birth, who now feels like a man
Transgender woman	Person with masculine sexual characteristics, identified as male at birth, who now feels like a woman
Gender Dysphoria/Gender Identity Disorder	Term used in DSM-V and ICD-10, respectively, to describe conditions by which gender nonconformity causes clinically significant distress or discomfort.
Transition	Time through which the person begins to live with a gender with which they identify, rather than with the gender assigned at birth
Real life experience	Full adoption of the gender role to which the person fits. This phase is necessary before the hormonalization processes and subsequent surgical body readjustment.
Drag queen	A man who dresses as a woman, usually for the purpose of entertainment or performance
Drag- king	A woman who dresses as a man, usually for the purpose of entertainment or performance
Shemale	Commonly used as a synonym for transgender. However, in some publications it is used to differentiate transgender people who have already undergone sexual readjustment processes.
Transvestism	Temporary foray into the clothing or accessories of the opposite sex for the purpose of sexual arousal and pleasure. It is considered a paraphilia

Table 1.
Definitions.

There is scarce and inaccurate information on the prevalence of transgender people in the general population; This is because population statistics reports exclude them, because trans people identify more with the denominations "man" or "woman" than with the identity of "trans," or because of the lack of inclusion of the "non-binary" category (neither masculine nor feminine) in the studies (**Table 1**) [11].

4. Social determinants for trans health

Social determinants of health are social and economic factors that influence people's lives and circumstances in ways that predispose them to certain health-related behaviors and health outcomes [12].

According to the WHO Commission on Determinants of Health, these determinants "*... are largely responsible for inequities in health—the unfair and avoidable health condition observed within and between countries*" and include factors such as social position, education, occupation, income, gender, and ethnicity/race.

The distribution of these factors has been empirically shown to correlate with how health problems are distributed across populations and within subpopulations. Addressing inequity in these factors would have multiple potential benefits in terms of better health and better life experiences and opportunities in general [13].

Increasingly, sexual orientation is recognized as a social determinant of health. Research has shown that sexual minorities are disproportionately affected by mental health problems, substance use problems, and HIV, compared with heterosexual populations globally [14].

A fundamental driver of health disparities for sexual minorities is sexual stigma, defined as "*negative regard, inferior status, and relative powerlessness that society collectively assigns to any non-heterosexual behavior, identity, relationship, or community.*" Sexual stigma influences health by causing unequal access to health services, psychological stress, and internal feelings of shame that influence health-related behavior [15].

The stigma associated with sexual orientation can also influence the social conditions and life opportunities available to sexual minorities. Access to these resources by sexual minorities is restricted because sexual stigma devalues people who are homosexual, bisexual, or who hold gender identities that do not conform to heterosexual norms [8, 9].

Restricted access to these resources can, in turn, influence "livelihood strategies," or the activities that people carry out and the decisions they make, in order to meet basic life needs such as food and shelter.

Transphobia plays a fundamental role as the determinant that conditions the health of people in this group.

5. Transphobia

Transphobia is "*the specific discrimination suffered by trans people since they put in question the prevailing sex/gender system from its roots, since they challenge the identity of gender assigned at birth*" [16].

Transphobia is etymologically a term of recent appearance, not yet included in the most current edition (2014) of the Dictionary of the Spanish Language of the Royal Spanish Academy (RAE). Despite this, the absence of an official description of a term does not imply its nonexistence. Continuing with the etymology, the word is made up of the particle "trans," which according to the RAE means "on the other side," and the word "phobia," which means "distressing and uncontrollable fear of certain acts, ideas, objects or situations, which it is known absurd and approaches the obsession" [17, 18].

Although according to this definition, we are faced with a fear that is supposed to be personal, arbitrary, and irrational, it is far from being so. This considered "phobia" has a much deeper root than a simple irrational fear, since it is anchored to a series of values and prejudices that we internalize when socializing in a certain culture [18].

Transphobia can manifest itself from subtle forms such as fear or negative beliefs, to much more explicit and aggressive forms such as intimidation, abuse, and even violence. There are two types of transphobia, direct and indirect. Indirect occurs when a supposedly neutral practice, rule, or criterion excludes or causes disadvantages either for reasons of gender identity, sexual orientation, or belonging to the LGTB group.

Direct transphobia consists of, for the reasons mentioned above, receiving less favorable treatment than another person who does not meet these characteristics and is in the same or equivalent situation [17].

Some noteworthy aspects in the activist and academic depathologizing discourses are the demand for recognition of both legal and health trans rights, the review of the healthcare model, and the questioning of the labels in the diagnostic classification manuals (ICD-10 and DSM) [18].

The controversy that is formed around this definition is wide, as well as the existing one about the psychiatric classification systems. This is due to the fact that, as we have commented and some authors explain, the deviation from the mean is considered abnormal, but frequently what is abnormal does not imply what is pathological. A clear example is homosexuality, excluded from the DSM in 1973 [19–21].

Thanks to activists and campaigns such as *Stop Trans Pathologization* (STP), these diagnostic manuals have adapted labels in order to abandon the psychopathological model that characterizes trans care.

The changes introduced in the DSM-V are still insufficient according to the STP, since the change of the title to "Gender Dysphoria" tries to reduce the stigma, but it is still debatable. For STP, this term associates the transition these people go through with a state of discomfort [9].

Although the terminological differences can be seen in the diagnostic criteria of last DSM speaks of "incongruence," which implies a "congruence" based on the normativity and pathologizes both transit and previous experiences. In addition, the criteria in the DSM-V require for their fulfillment that the person shows at least two of those described in the figure, during a period of 6 months or more [19].

As for ICD-10, the term "Transsexualism" is found within Mental and Behavioral Disorders, while in ICD-11 we find a new chapter called "Conditions related to sexual health", where the "Discordance of gender" in adults, adolescents. and infants.

Other barriers include: financial barriers (lack of insurance, lack of income), discrimination, lack of cultural competency by healthcare providers, health systems barriers (electronic records, forms, lab referrals, inappropriate clinical facilities), and socioeconomic barriers (transportation, housing, mental health). While other minority groups face some of these healthcare barriers, many are unique, and many are significantly magnified for transgender people [22].

6. Situation of the trans population in Paraguay

Paraguay has ratified numerous international instruments for the protection of human rights, by which it is obliged to adopt measures to guarantee the sexual and reproductive health of all people and nondiscrimination based on sex, sexual orientation, and gender identity.

The amount of information referring to this situation in the country is scarce.

Regarding the development of guarantees and rights in the matter, our legal framework is manifested in the following ways:

The National Constitution of Paraguay (1992) states [23]:

- **ARTICLE 24 - RELIGIOUS AND IDEOLOGICAL FREEDOM**

Religious freedom, worship and ideology are recognized, with no other limitations than those established in this Constitution and in the law. No confession will have an official character.

The independence and autonomy of churches and religious denominations are guaranteed, with no other limitations than those imposed in this Constitution and the laws.

Nobody can be bothered, investigated or forced to testify because of their beliefs or their ideology.

- **ARTICLE 25 - EXPRESSION OF PERSONALITY**

Every person has the right to free expression of their personality, creativity and the formation of their own identity and image.

Ideological pluralism is guaranteed.

- **ARTICLE 46 - EQUALITY OF PEOPLE**

All the inhabitants of the Republic are equal in dignity and rights. Discrimination is not allowed. The State will remove the obstacles and prevent the factors that maintain or promote them.

The protections that are established on unfair inequalities will not be considered as discriminatory factors but rather as egalitarian.

- **ARTICLE 68 - RIGHT TO HEALTH**

The State shall protect and promote health as a fundamental right of the person and in the interest of the community.

No one shall be deprived of public assistance to prevent or treat diseases, pests or plagues, and relief in the event of catastrophes and accidents.

Every person is obliged to submit to the sanitary measures established by law, while respecting human dignity.

It is recognized that sex work is the main economic activity of 86% of trans people, although it is work that is not punished in Paraguay, but it is also not recognized or regulated by law. Access to jobs is impeded by discrimination due to the fact of assuming a different sexual identity, since transgender people are not hired in private entities, except in hairdressing salons or volunteering in the field of health [24].

Working life is further complicated by the fact that more than half (52%) of transgender people did not complete primary school and ended up dropping out of school due to the "*teasing, harassment, physical punishment and degrading treatment*" they received from other students and teachers [25].

Transgender encounter the same degrading treatment when they go to health services, where they are subjected to psychological aggression and humiliation when they require health care in general, and especially when they go to obtain treatment and care for HIV and AIDS.

According to the Ministry of Public Health and Social Welfare of Paraguay (MSPyBS), in the general population, the prevalence of HIV infection (2017) was 23% in this population. The cascade of the continuum of HIV care in 2019 in the population of trans women shows that, for the period cited, there are 187 (96.4%) people alive who know their diagnosis, are on ART 114 (58.8%).

Lastly, 63 (32.5%) of people living with HIV have their viral load suppressed, representing a gap of 67.5%. In this case, the pillar of diagnosed trans women is practically saturated, and the main difficulty is observed in the low percentage of trans women who maintain a suppressed viral load. It can be concluded that some type of barrier must exist to ensure that this population group maintains adherence to antiretroviral treatment [26].

6.1 Paraguayan health regulations for the trans population

Regarding the Regulations, in Paraguay Resolution No. 72/2012, of the General Directorate of Penitentiary Establishments and Criminal Enforcement of the Ministry of Justice, "*Which establishes new regulations for the operation of the benefit of private visits in penitentiaries and correctional facilities for women of the Republic.*" Among these, neither the sex nor the gender of the visiting partner of the person deprived of liberty is determined [27].

In addition to this, in 2015, the Protocol for Attention to Trans Persons Deprived of Liberty was established. On the part of the MSPyBS, through Resolution No. 695/2016, the use of the social name for trans people is recommended [28].

This is why determining the knowledge and biases of the existing medical workforce should be included: medical students, physicians in training, practicing physicians, and other health workers across the spectrum of training; the adequacy of enough providers for the care required, and the state of a framework for paying for adequate care.

There is a specific need to determine if providers receive adequate training in transgender medicine and, if not, determine the gap. There is also a specific need to determine the current state of discrimination against transgender people in the health-care system. Additionally, studies should determine possible solutions to address gaps (including training for knowledge gaps and policy changes for financial gaps) along with mechanisms to validate such solutions.

7. Discussion

This population faces a series of problems to access health services in their countries, and Paraguay is no exception, many of the situations are linked to stigmatization, lack of medical care protocols, and lack of information on how to act in certain situations, which is determined by the lack of inclusion in the training curricula of health professionals [12, 25, 26].

Although the health problems that affect transgender people are similar to those that affect the rest of the population, some conditions are more widespread within these groups because they face situations that increase their vulnerability or risk of exposure to pathogens [1, 6].

Different studies indicate that they are mostly affected by infectious diseases such as HIV, syphilis, gonorrhea, hepatitis, or genital herpes, to mention a few examples [7].

The first challenge that trans people face, and the one that permeates almost all the other challenges, is the one that has to do with the adequate recognition of their identities, and the fight for the reduction of transphobia, for the purposes of offering comprehensive and quality care [8].

There is also a great lack of education in all the staff, about their realities and rights; as well as the appropriate care protocols since there are women with a penis and men with a vulva, who require different treatments and accompaniments to achieve the full enjoyment of their identities, these points must be discussed by decision-makers in order to help the inclusion of all groups within the health service. Although, in Paraguay, the use of the social name can be found, discrimination and stigmatization continue to be an important problem [10–13].

In the development of trans identities, acceptance is an aspect that perhaps has the most serious consequences for the health and full development of all the rights of these people. Although the medicalization of their bodies and sexualities has existed since the nineteenth century, due to the fact that all their diverse expressions were marginalized and cataloged by scientific discourse as abnormal and disturbed, requiring medical intervention to undo everything that does not fit into the imposed ideal dichotomy [14, 26].

An important point to note is also that 39% of the transgender population suffers from serious psychological distress (compared with 5% of the general population) that they have a nine times higher risk of suicide attempts and a five times higher frequency of infection for HIV (mostly transgender women), 25% did not seek medical care for fear of mistreatment in care services, which is striking due to the constant increase [25–27].

Violence motivated by sexual orientation or gender in sexual minorities indicates the presence of 68% of physical violence inflicted and 49% of sexual violence [15], in Paraguay there is a lack of studies that can demonstrate the real impact of transphobia in services of health and in addition to this study on the burden of diseases and disorders.

The limitations of this review are based on the scarcity of studies to carry out the study, so it is suggested to carry out a study to provide evidence on the health of trans people in Paraguay.

8. Conclusions

In conclusion, it is highlighted that although Paraguay has ratified numerous international instruments for the protection of human rights, there is still a lack of measures to guarantee the sexual and reproductive health of all people and nondiscrimination based on sex, sexual orientation, and gender identity.

In addition to public policies aimed at this group, it is necessary to establish gender regulations or laws that allow the population to develop in an integral manner.

Conflict of interest

The authors declare no conflict of interest.

Author details

Carlos Miguel Rios-González[1,2,3]

1 Faculty of Medical Sciences, National University of Caaguazu, Paraguay

2 Ministry of Public Health and Social Welfare, National Institute of Health, Asunción, Paraguay

3 South American University, Pedro Juan Caballero, Paraguay

*Address all correspondence to: carlosmigue_rios@live.com

References

[1] IOM (Institute of Medicine). The Health of Lesbian, Gay, Bisexual, and Transgender People: Building a Foundation for Better Understanding. Washington, DC: The National Academies Press; 2011

[2] Council of Europe. Commissioner for Human Rights. Strasbourg: Council of Europe; 2015

[3] European Union Agency for Fundamental Rights (FRA). The Fundamental Rights Situation of Intersex People. 2015. Available from: https://fra.europa.eu/en/publication/2015/fundamental-rights-situation-intersex-people

[4] World Health Organization (WHO). Eliminating Forced, Coercive and Otherwise Involuntary Sterilization: An Interagency Statement. Geneva, Switzerland: OHCHR, UN Women, UNAIDS, UNDP, UNFPA, UNICEF and WHO; 2014

[5] Reisner SL, Poteat T, Keatley J, Cabral M, Mothopeng T, Dunham E, et al. Global health burden and needs of transgender populations: A review. Lancet. 2016;**388**(10042):412-436

[6] Barrington C, Wejnert C, Guardado ME, Nieto AL, Bailey GP. Social network characteristics and HIV vulnerability among transgender persons in San Salvador: Identifying opportunities for HIV prevention strategies. AIDS and Behavior. 2012;**16**(1):214-224

[7] Andrinopoulos K, Hembling J, Guardado ME, de Maria Hernández F, Nieto AI, Melendez G. Evidence of the negative effect of sexual minority stigma on HIV testing among MSM and transgender women in San Salvador, El Salvador. AIDS and Behavior. 2015;**19**(1):60-71. DOI: 10.1007/s10461-014-0813-0

[8] Suess SA. Trans health care from a depathologization and human rights perspective. Public Health Reviews. 2020;**41**(1):1-17

[9] Hanssmann C. Epidemiological rage: Population, biography, and state responsibility in trans-health activism. Social Science & Medicine. 2020;**247**:112808

[10] Schwend AS. The trans depathologization perspective: A contribution to public health approaches and clinical practices in mental health? SESPAS Report 2020. Gaceta sanitaria. 2020;**34**:54-60

[11] T'Sjoen G, Arcelus J, De Vries AL, Fisher AD, Nieder TO, Özer M, et al. European Society for Sexual Medicine position statement "Assessment and hormonal management in adolescent and adult trans people, with attention for sexual function and satisfaction". The Journal of Sexual Medicine. 2020;**17**(4):570-584

[12] Davies C, Elder CV, Riggs DW, Robinson KH. The importance of informed fertility counselling for trans young people. The Lancet Child & Adolescent Health. 2021;**5**(9):e36-e37

[13] Bouman WP, Schwend AS, Motmans J, Smiley A, Safer JD, Deutsch MB, et al. Language and trans health. International Journal of Transgenderism. 2017;**18**(1):1-6

[14] Giffort DM, Underman K. The relationship between medical education and trans health disparities: A call to research. Sociology Compass. 2016;**10**(11):999-1013

[15] Wagner PE, Kunkel A, Asbury MB, Soto F. Health (trans) gressions: Identity and stigma management in trans* healthcare support seeking. Women & Language. 2016;**39**(1):49-74

[16] Lombardi E. Public health and trans-people: Barriers to care and strategies to improve treatment. In: The Health of Sexual Minorities. Boston, MA: Springer; 2007. pp. 638-652

[17] Jaspal R, Nambiar KZ, Delpech V, Tariq S. HIV and trans and non-binary people in the UK. Sexually Transmitted Infections. 2018;**94**(5):318-319

[18] Zeeman L, Sherriff N, Browne K, McGlynn N, Mirandola M. A review of lesbian, gay, bisexual, trans and intersex (LGBTI) health and healthcare inequalities. European Journal of Public Health. 2019;**29**(5):974-980

[19] World Health Organization (WHO). Sexual Health, Human Rights and the Law. Geneva, Switzerland: World Health Organization; 2015

[20] Valenzuela AV, Velásquez RC. Salud comunitaria, la experiencia de salud trans en el Servicio de Salud Talcahuano. Chile. Psicoperspectivas. 2020;**19**(2):153-165

[21] Coleman E, Botzer M, Cohen-Kettenis P, De Cuypere G, Feldman J, et al. Normas de Atención para la salud de personas trans y con variabilidad de género: La Asociación Mundial para la Salud Transgénero. International Journal of Transgenderism. 2018;**19**(3):287-354

[22] De Benedictis-Serrano GA, Rios-González CM. The LGBT community and HIV: An incorrect medical judgment. Travel Medicine and Infectious Disease. 2018;**25**:18-19. DOI: 10.1016/j.tmaid.2018.04.017

[23] Restar A, Jin H, Operario D. Gender-inclusive and gender-specific approaches in trans health research. Transgender Health. 2021;**6**(5):235-239

[24] Constitución Nacional de la Republica del Paraguay. 2022. Available from: https://www.bacn.gov.py/leyes-paraguayas/9580/constitucion-nacional

[25] Ortiz-Martínez Y, Ríos-González CM. Need for more research on and health interventions for transgender people. Sexual Health. 2017 Apr;**14**(2):196-197. DOI: 10.1071/SH16148

[26] Aguilar G, Samudio T, Lopez G, Jimenez L, Wilson EC, McFarland W, et al. High HIV prevalence among transgender women in Paraguay. International Journal of STD & AIDS. 2020 Nov;**31**(13):1308-1314

[27] Ministerio de Justicia. Resolución N.° 72/2012. 2022. Available from: https://codehupy.org.py/ddhh2020/wp-content/uploads/2020/12/IGUALDAD-LGTBI__WEB.pdf

[28] Ministerio de Salud Publica y Bienestar Social. Resolución N.° 695/2016. 2022. Available from: http://www.panambi.org.py/noticias/detalle/132/Las+personas+Trans+podr%C3%A1n+utilizar+su+nombre+social+en+cl%C3%ADnicas.++

Section 3

Advances and New Perspectives

Chapter 6

Standards Developments for Improving Care for Transgender People

Kelly Davison

Abstract

Outdated GSSO information practices contribute to institutional and interpersonal stigma for transgender people in healthcare. Poorly defined data elements, conflated sex and gender concepts, constrained representation of gender variation, and lack of cultural understanding on the part of health information professionals and clinicians are contributing to healthcare environments and interactions that stigmatize transgender people and that drive health inequities. In this chapter, I will review recent developments in standards oriented toward addressing gender bias in the technical structures that support healthcare institutions. I will focus on the international work of Canada Health Infoway's Sex and Gender Working Group and the Health Level Seven International Gender Harmony Project. The intent is to provide an overview of these efforts and garner further interest, participation and adoption standards that support safe and gender-affirming healthcare for all people.

Keywords: GSSO information practices, Canada Health Infoway, Sex and Gender Working Group, HL7 International, Gender Harmony Model, health equity

1. Introduction

An estimated 1–3% of people in Canada are transgender, and just over 7% of Canadians identify as lesbian, gay or bisexual [1]. Approximately 32% of them report having unmet healthcare needs [2]. In the United States, there are over 1,000,000 transgender people, a third of which report avoiding healthcare for fear of discrimination [3]. Transgender people and sex and gender minorities (SGM) experience unnecessary and preventable health inequities including higher rates of mortality, depression, anxiety, substance use, chronic disease and suicidality which are, in part, the summary result of atrocious experiences of discrimination and stigmatization on the part of healthcare staff and institutions [1, 4–6]. Institutionalized cisheteronormativity, a term which refers to the culturally-driven normalization of cisgender, heterosexual status and the invisibilization of non-cis, non-heterosexual people [7, 8], is a primary social bias encoded into digital health structures and care cultures that prevents meaningful knowledge development about the health status and needs of this population [1, 6, 7]. Poorly defined data elements, conflated sex and gender concepts, constrained representation of gender variation, and lack of cultural understanding on the part of health information professionals and clinicians are all conditions contributing to healthcare systems, environments and interactions that stigmatize transgender people, and that drive health inequities [1, 6–10]. Since 2019, technical, data and messaging standards development organizations (SDOs) have been working to modernize gender, sex and sexual orientation (GSSO) information practices in electronic health records (EHRs) to enable inclusive and affirming care for transgender people and SGM [1, 8, 11]. In this chapter, I will provide an overview of these recent innovations, including work of Canada Health Infoway's Sex and Gender Working Group and the HL7 Gender Harmony Model.

1.1 Health is a human right

The global population of transgender people and SGM live with higher burdens of disease and lower health than many other populations, especially cisgender people [12, 13]. Despite of the fact that the human rights of transgender people are protected by national and internal law [14], transgender people continue to face severe discrimination. The experiences of transgender people in healthcare, at the hands of healthcare staff, are atrocious [1], and ought to be a central concern to healthcare decision makers, policy makers and legal supports, and to society at large [15, 16]. Healthcare, as an organizational, regional, national and global social system with a specific ethical orientation that ought to adhere to, uphold, and advocate for the Universal Human Rights of transgender people, and *Health for All* [17]. Health is a human right [18]. Modernization of outdated gender, sex and sexual orientation information practices is a foundational step to creating healthcare institutions that are gender-affirming [9, 10, 12, 13].

2. Outdated GSSO information practices

Modernization of outdated GSSO information practices is an equity-oriented endeavor [19] intended to address the technical conditions that enable structural and institutional bias and that contribute to health inequities for transgender people and SGM [16]. Information practices include the definition, collection, organization, sharing and use of health information [17]. The term "Gender, Sex and Sexual Orientation" or "GSSO" was coined by C. Kronk, PhD of Yale University, who has created and published a Queer Ontology to facilitate increased awareness and improved understanding and consistency of use of GSSO terms [14, 20]. Outdated GSSO information practices include:

- Poor definition of GSSO information
- Conflation of the meaning of distinct gender and sex concepts.
- Problems related to collection of GSSO information
- Confusion as to who should be collecting what GSSO information, when, and for what purpose(s) in healthcare workflows.
- Problems related to the organization of GSSO information

- Use of sex and gender codes as though they are interchangeable and synonymous in administrative and clinical domains.
- Problems related to information sharing and exchange
- Problematic mapping of sex and gender codes between code systems in exchange standards.
- Inadequate representation of sex and gender diversity in exchange standards.
- Problems of use
- Unconscious bias and assumptions related to sex and gender concepts.
- Inadequate emphasis on quality clinical care and the therapeutic relationship for SGM.
- Overemphasis on business requirements and efficiency at the expense of clinical care quality.

3. Modernizing GSSO information practices

Building on the momentum of the work of such expert agencies as the Fenway Institute, Trans Care BC and Rainbow Health Ontario, there has been a recent increase in activity related to raising the critical awareness about the importance of diversity, equity, and the role of healthcare in creating the conditions for the well health of transgender people and SGM in North America and beyond [11, 12]. A diverse international community of people and organizations, including expert agencies, SDOs, researchers, EHR and solutions vendors, healthcare professionals and health information professionals, have dedicated their time and expertise to making healthcare more inclusive. In this section, I will discuss key developments within this community and key activities in relation to the healthcare of transgender people and SGM beginning with my own country, Canada.

3.1 Canada Health Infoway

Heading up the co-development, maintenance and support of technical and interoperability standards that support healthcare in the country, Canada Health Infoway (Infoway) has been a key organization enabling digital health in Canada since 2001. As Canada's National Release Center for such technical standards as the HL7 International information exchange standards, the Systematized Nomenclature of Medicine—Clinical Terms (SNOMED CT) and Logical Observation Identifiers, Names and Codes (LOINC), Infoway's mandate includes bringing a Canadian perspective to international standards development with SDOs such as HL7 International, SNOMED International, and the Regenstrief Institute. At the national level, Infoway collaborates with a network of pan-Canadian Healthcare Organizations, provinces, jurisdictions, vendors and governance bodies to support the implementation of technical standards in the Canadian digital health ecosystem and develops, maintains and publishes pan-Canadian and jurisdictional subsets via the Terminology Gateway service. Infoway convenes stakeholders by establishing communities for collaboration and working groups on a central information sharing and engagement platform, InfoCentral. One such working group is Infoway's Sex and Gender Working Group (SGWG).

3.2 Canada Health Infoway's sex and gender working group

Infoway's SGWG was established in 2019 with the primary aim of modernizing outdated GSSO information practices in Canadian electronic health records [17] to support the health of all Canadians. Since then, this international community of researchers, pan-Canadian Health Organizations, healthcare agency representatives, subject matter experts, and people with lived experience have been convening monthly to share recent and relevant research, discuss the process of modernization [17] and lead modernization by taking evidence-informed action.

3.3 A proposed action plan to modernize GSSO information practices

After 2 years of convening, Infoway's Sex-Gender Working Group produced *A Proposed Action Plan to Modernize GSSO Information Practices in Canadian Electronic Health Records* (the Action Plan) in early 2021 [17]. This visionary work, led by Dr. Francis Lau of the University of Victoria and supported by a network of people and agencies participating in the SGWG including Health Canada, the Canadian Institutes of Health Research Institute of Gender and Health, Canada Health Infoway, the Canadian Institute for Health Information, the Canadian Health Information Management Association, the University of Victoria GSSO research team and more, provides a comprehensive summary of existing research and proposes a plan to modernize the outdated GSSO information practices that stigmatize transgender people and SGM [21]. Although grounded in the grassroots of Canadian healthcare, the vision, recommendations and research knowledge outlined the Action Plan could be applied internationally. There are seven primary aims of the GSSO Action Plan produced by the Infoway SGWG:

1. Envisage an equity- and SGM-oriented health system that embraces diversity and aligns with other SGM-related initiatives.

2. Engage organizations and communities across Canada to modernize GSSO information practices in EHRs that support equity-oriented healthcare and meet SGM needs.

3. Establish a precise, inclusive, appropriate, evolving and multi-level GSSO terminology with standardized data definitions, coding schemes and value sets to support affirming patient care, provide complete and accurate health system use of data and inform health research.

4. Adopt a common set of EHR functions that support the collection and use of standardized GSSO data, SGM-oriented clinical care guidelines (e.g. radiation shielding in imaging exams, cancer screening, lab reference ranges, reminders, and reports), clinical quality improvement, data-driven analytics, health system performance tracking and health evidence generation.

5. Integrate and tailor GSSO data collection and use including secondary uses within all organizational structures, policies, practices, governance, use cases and workflow processes in order to be responsive to specific care needs of SGM.

6. Educate and train healthcare staff to enhance their capacity to provide culturally competent and safe care, and implementers, policy makers and researchers to ensure required safeguards in place to protect these data. Inform patients on the need for GSSO data collection and protections for safe access and use.

7. Establish a central hub to liaise, guide, assist and monitor the progress of this action plan over time [21].

Although there remains much work to do, members of Infoway's SGWG are using the Action Plan and its aims as a guide to specify and cultivate adoption of modern, consensus-based data, technical and exchange standards that address structural cisheternormativity in Canadian healthcare. The community continues to meet on a monthly basis and drive new research, insights, and the development of modern approaches and practices to realize the aims outlined in the Action Plan.

The continued support of standards organizations such as Canada Health Infoway will play a foundational role in the ongoing process of modernization of healthcare. More information about Canada Health Infoway and Infoway Communities can be found on InfoCentral.

4. HL7 International

The beliefs, attitudes and organizational practices required to create culturally and psychologically safe, quality healthcare for transgender people will be adopted by individual health organizations. However, meaningful change will not happen unless the standards that we use to communicate health information from one service to another—the standards we use to connect a continuum of care services—are also modernized such that they are inclusive of transgender people and SGM and are designed to address the problems related to outdated information practices. Health information exchange standards (sometimes referred to as messaging standards) are powerful drivers of systemic change. As a world-leading exchange standard development organization, HL7 International plays an important role in the specification and implementation of health information exchange standards that support *Health for All*.

4.1 The HL7 International gender harmony project

In 2019, HL7 International created the Gender Harmony Project as an open, international collaboration of volunteers and experts from international agencies and SDOs dedicated to creating gender-inclusive standards in healthcare, and to addressing harms associated with biased exchange standards [11]. Members of this group have been meeting regularly to define, specify, model and explicate the Gender Harmony Logical Model since its establishment.

4.2 The HL7 International gender harmony logical model

In early 2021, the Gender Harmony Project produced the informative-ballot-for-comment that outlines the Gender Harmony Logical Model. Input on the document was collected from international stakeholders, and the first release of the informative document was published by the HL7 International Vocabulary Working Group in August of 2021: *Gender Harmony—Modeling Sex and Gender Representation, Release 1* [22]. The Gender Harmony Logical Model is a model that can be applied in the design of inclusive digital health systems and messaging standards such as HL7 version 2 (HL7v2), Version 3 (V3), Clinical Document Architecture (CDA®) and Fast Health Interoperability Resources (FHIR®) used to exchange health information between digital health systems [11]. The Gender Harmony Logical Model supports modernized design of interoperable EHRs and related standards, and is designed to enable:

4.2.1 Improved definition of gender and sex information

1. Unambiguous, evidence and consensus-based definitions of key sex and gender concepts that support model elements.

2. Avoidance of stigmatization in value sets by enabling nonbinary options without the use of such labels as "other" or "complex" in model elements.

4.2.2 Improved guidance on collection of gender and sex information

- Explicit description of model concept and element attributes means that organization of administrative and clinical GSSO information is clearly defined, streamlining GSSO data collection use cases.

4.2.3 Clear organization of gender and sex information

1. Clear definition of administrative and clinical sex and gender data.

2. Clear division between administrative and clinical sex and gender data in model elements.

3. Clear articulation of essential elements that support affirmative care interactions.

4.2.4 Semantic sharing and exchange

1. Unambiguously defined concepts and clear organization of model element concepts and attributes reduces risk for transformation of sex and gender concepts during sharing and exchange.

2. Representation of gender diversity in messaging standards.

4.2.5 Reduced risk of use of outdated information practices

1. Reduces unconscious bias and unchecked assumptions related to sex and gender.

2. Emphasizes care quality by supporting gender-affirming patient-provider interactions.

3. Supports business requirements by separating administrative data from clinical data.

The consistent application of the Gender Harmony Model in the design of joined-up health information systems is a shift in paradigms—from outdated GSSO information practices to modern ones, and a shift that enables quality healthcare for transgender people and SGM.

4.3 The gender harmony paradigm

The Gender Harmony Paradigm in healthcare is implementing systems design that addresses conditions resulting in health inequities for SGM. It involves meaningful integration of the HL7 Gender Harmony Logical Model, modern GSSO information practices and associated standards enabling culturally safer institutional policies and practices that support inclusive healthcare for transgender and SGM people. The Gender Harmony Model reduces real and latent harms associated with current gender constructs in health by: (1) decoupling administrative and clinical concepts in digital health systems; (2) addressing the conditions that lead to negative clinical interactions that deter transgender people from seeking care (e.g. being misgendered, misnamed or outed); and finally (3) by addressing conditions that make transgender people and people with nonbinary gender identities invisible to clinicians, policy makers, analysts and researchers who use health information for system improvement. At the patient level, the Gender Harmony Model enables clinicians' use of person-centred language in clinical interactions and provides them with the information necessary for objective and appropriate preventive screening, treatment and referral options based on unambiguous sex and gender health information. At the organizational level, implementation of the Gender Harmony Model involves the adoption and use of logical, technical and data standards necessary to support gender affirming care cultures and practices. At the health system level, implementation of the model orients clinical and institutional healthcare toward gender equity by addressing problems associated with the omission of data elements required to generate knowledge for health system improvement.

4.4 HL7 International gender harmony model overview

The Gender Harmony Logical Model, which I will call 'the Model' throughout the remainder of this chapter for ease of reading, does not exclusively benefit transgender and nonbinary people. All patients benefit from higher quality care and analytics enabled by the Model. Application of the Model can broadly be considered a step toward personalized medicine and more person-centred care since it enables more granular use and understanding of complex social and medical phenomena. The data elements of the Model [22] are designed to address the conditions that are currently leading to health inequities for transgender people such as problems associated with omission of data elements required for affirming care (i.e. Name to Use, Pronouns), conflation of administrative sex and gender concepts (i.e. Gender Identity, Recorded Sex or Gender) and by creating opportunities for clinicians to provide care by specifying care needs, rather than making assumptions related to outdated binary constructs (i.e. Sex for Clinical Use) [11]. In this section, I will provide an overview of each data element and its specific attributes that support design and implementation decisions in digital health systems such as EHRs. Model data elements will be capitalized to improve readability.

4.4.1 Gender identity

In healthcare, knowing a patient's gender identity allows clinicians to provide informed and affirming, quality care, without misgendering them based on assumptions or pre-existing and out of date information in the patient record. All people have a gender identity. Gender Identity is a person or patient's personal sense of being a man, woman, boy, girl or something else [22]. Gender identity must be declared by the person or patient, rather than them being labeled with it. Gender identity is fluid and can change, and so must be collected routinely [23]. People can identify with none, one, or many genders, and can set time constraints on specific gender identities. Gender Identity should be used in conjunction with the other Model data elements to support gender-affirming, quality healthcare and should be validated privately with the patient to avoid outing them. Outing is when information about a person's gender or sexual identity is made known to specific people without permission. If this is done by a clerk or a clinician in the context of an emergency room or a waiting room, it may be directly harmful to the person being outed or lead to harm. As with all EHR data, informed consent about collection, sharing and use of Gender Identity information should be acquired before it is entered in the patient chart.

In order to ensure international applicability of the Model, the terms *male gender identity* and *female gender identity* have been used to represent gender identities associated with binary male and female sexes. The term nonbinary gender identity is proposed as a value option to represent code value options that are not accurately represented within the binary male/female construct [22].

Gender Identity is included in the Canadian Institute for Health Information CIHI Reference Data Model [24] (CRDM) and the United States Core Data for Interoperability Version 2 [25] (USCDIv2).

4.4.2 Name to use

Name to Use is the name that the person accessing healthcare services uses and wishes the care team to use. Importantly, Name to Use may not simply be a person's preferred name. Name to Use may be a name associated with the person's gender identity, and so should be used in healthcare interactions to avoid misnaming or outing people. Name to Use may or may not be consistent with a person's legal name. Misnaming people based on legal records can be harmful, so it is best to ensure that the name the patient uses is validated privately, and that this validated information is updated in the patient record routinely and promptly upon patient arrival to prevent misnaming or outing in subsequent care interactions. Use of the Name to Use may be time-limited [22].

4.4.3 Pronouns

Pronouns (also called third person pronouns, personal pronouns and incorrectly often called preferred pronouns) and possessives are language tools used to communicate with and about people. They include such options as he/him/his, she/her/

hers, and they/them/theirs, among many options [7]. Pronouns come in sets. The most common pronouns used are gendered, and so by validating pronouns used by a patient and updating the care record before clinical interactions occur, intake staff can help ensure that patients are not misgendered by clinicians in subsequent interactions by the use of incorrect pronouns, and maintain the integrity of the therapeutic relationship. The Pronouns data element of the Model complements Gender Identity and Name to Use to ensure that communications with and about a patient are person-centred and affirming of their gender [21]. A useful rule of thumb is that until pronouns are confirmed by the patient, the gender-neutral options they/them/theirs can be used in interpersonal interactions to avoid misgendering. Like Name to Use and Gender Identity, patients may use more than one pronoun or set of pronouns, and their use of specific pronouns may be time delimited.

4.4.4 Recorded sex or gender

One of the primary problems associated with outdated GSSO information practices is that sex and gender concepts, the code values that represent them, the labels on the data fields they occupy and their distinct meanings, are conflated and used as though they are synonymous [6]. Administrative values cannot be used for clinical decision making with 100% reliability, particularly when used in the care of people whose sex at birth does not align with their gender identity and people who identify as transgender. Separating the sex or gender value that has been recorded on identification and other administrative or legal artifacts from clinical sex and gender identity helps to reduce unchecked assumptions about anatomy based on inaccurate recorded sex or gender information. The Model data element called Recorded Sex or Gender does just this: it separates administrative sex and gender information from the clinical sex and gender information, and is necessary to provide safe, quality, and gender-affirming clinical interactions.

Because there are so many different possibilities in the documentation that patients can present to support identification, it may be important to know the provenance of the Recorded Sex or Gender information. Provenance includes details about the jurisdiction that issued the record, its acquisition date, its validity period, and information about the source record including the name and definition of the field name and definition. Sex or gender information that is displayed on drivers' licenses, government IDs, birth certificates and other documents are Recorded Sex or Gender information. In many cases, this information is acquired through active interfaces between health information systems and government administrative databases via exchange standards. Inconsistencies between Recorded Sex or Gender data values and Gender Identity should not automatically be regarded as erroneous and should be validated with the patient.

Birth sex, or sex assigned at birth, as an example of recorded sex or gender that is present in most care records, is included in the CRDM [24] and the USCDIv2 [25].

4.4.5 Sex for clinical use

Sex for Clinical Use is a novel clinical data element that supports person-centred care by enabling clinicians to specify clinical sex beyond binary options based on different observations. Much like the explicit inclusion of a patient-declared Gender Identity, the key value of Sex for Clinical Use is that it enables the removal of unchecked assumptions about a person's sex that may be present in administrative binary male/female constructs. To achieve this, a provider may refer to an anatomic inventory, a surgical history, a hormonal inventory or other artifacts that inform the context for the observation. Four such examples include:

- ordering a screening mammography for a transman who has had top surgery;
- specifying testicular protection for a transgender woman receiving an imaging procedure;
- referencing a nonbinary hormonal reference range for a nonbinary person in transition; or
- ordering a Pap smear for a man whose sex assigned at birth does not match his gender identity.

Full transition is not always required to address gender dysphoria [10], but the ability for providers to reduce unchecked assumptions based on recorded sex or gender, and provide agile, appropriate and quality care to all people is an important feature that the model supports. Value options that are proposed for the model include 'male,' 'female' and 'specified' sex for clinical use. The term 'specified' was chosen for the Model to eliminate stigma associated with a value options of 'complex' (not all patients who may benefit from the use of this element are particularly complex), to align with the use case where an option is specified by the provider, and to enable backwards compatibility with (and avoid use) of the stigmatizing term 'other,' as is so commonly used in health information systems [8].

5. Stigma, encoded

When used together, the five data elements of the Gender Harmony Logical Model facilitate the tight alignment between social concepts, code systems, health terminology standards, exchange standards, EHR design and healthcare practices required to address stigma and drive health equity through the provision of gender-affirming care. However, code systems and health terminology standards are dynamic in nature and remain prone to the inappropriate codification of stigmatizing or pathologizing terms, codes or concepts [4]. As society becomes more complex and technology become more ubiquitous, the importance of remaining vigilant for standards that exclude marginalized populations and intersectional patient identities will become increasingly important. Primary care providers, in particular, are instrumental to the implementation of changes that will close the equity gap for transgender people because they provide the bulk of preventive screening and treatment related care and serve as a primary coordination point for patients. Modernized GSSO information practices help primary care providers to ensure that patients are appropriately matched to their care needs, and that assumptions related to conflated sex and gender concepts are avoided [13]. However, regulated health information professionals that have healthcare-specific training and awareness of healthcare models, ethics and practice will play a critical role in supporting modernization efforts. Certified Terminology Standards Specialists (CTSS), Certified Classification and Coding Specialist (CCCS), Certified Healthcare Information Management (CHIM) professional credentials, signal professional adherence to a base set of demonstrated competencies and ethics, and professionals with health information credentials such as these are more likely to have knowledge about the importance of the therapeutic relationship and downstream impacts of technical design on patient care [26]. A major responsibility of certified health information professionals is to align technical design with clinical requirements such that the integrity of this most sacred and fundamental component of healthcare—the therapeutic relationship—is protected. Like credentialed and regulated clinicians, certified health information professionals are accountable for upholding the core evidence-based values and ethics that support healthcare (i.e., person-centred care, trauma-informed care, the Gender Harmony Logical Model). The Digital Health Revolution has arrived [27], and the ongoing datafication of healthcare and society means that informatics professionals must regularly visit their ethics to ensure they are aligned with healthcare values, develop critical awareness of the impact of structural bias in data and technical design and standards on social justice, cultivate ethical communities around the design and analysis of information systems and standards, and evaluate the impact of their work on the lives of the patients they serve [28].

6. Conclusion

Transgender people experience unnecessary and preventable health inequities that are, in part, the result of social bias encoded into the technical and data structures that connect systems in the digital health ecosystem. Poorly defined data elements, conflated sex and gender concepts, constrained representation of gender variation in code systems, outdated terminology standards and health information exchange standards contribute to this harm. Canada Health Infoway's Sex and Gender Working Group is an international, transdisciplinary community of people and agencies with an Action Plan to modernize gender, sex and sexual orientation information practices in healthcare. The HL7 International Gender Harmony Project has recently published the first release of the informative document for the Gender Harmony Logical Model, a consensus-based, evidence-informed logical model developed to address outdated information practices and support the modernization of healthcare for sex and gender minorities. Though there remains much work to do, this dedicated international community of professionals, researchers and people with lived experience are undertaking actions that enable inclusive and affirming care for transgender people and SGM.

Acknowledgements

I gratefully acknowledge the ongoing support of these efforts by Health Canada, Canada Health Infoway, all the members, agencies and presenters participating in Infoway's Sex-Gender Working Group, the Canadian Institute of Health Information, the Canadian Health Information Management Association, the Office of the National Coordinator, HL7 Canada, HL7 International and the University of Victoria GSSO Research Team, the Canadian Institutes for Health Research, Michael Smith Health Research BC, the Community-Based Research Centre, and the large community of people, providers and agencies dedicated to equitable health for transgender people and sex and gender minorities for their continued work toward a better humanity, and a better future.

Conflict of interest

The author(s) declare no conflict of interest.

Notes/thanks/other declarations

My thanks to Dr. Francis Lau for his review of this chapter as I was drafting it. The information provided in this chapter has been derived from my participation as Co-Chair in Infoway's Sex and Gender Working Group and participation in the HL7 Gender Harmony Project. Please report any mistakes or inconsistencies to me at kdaviso@uvic.ca

Author details

Kelly Davison
University of Victoria, Victoria, British Columbia, Canada

*Address all correspondence to: kdaviso@uvic.ca

References

[1] Canadian House of Commons Standing Committee on Health. Committee report: The health of LGBTQIA2 communities in Canada [Internet]. Casey B, editor. The Parliament of Canada; 2019. Available from: https://www.ourcommons.ca/DocumentViewer/en/42-1/HESA/report-28/

[2] Giblon R, Bauer GR. Healthcare availability, quality, and unmet need: A comparison of transgender and cisgender residents of Ontario, Canada. BMC Health Services Research. 2017;**17**(1):283

[3] Kronk CA, Everhart AR, Ashley F, Thompson HM, Schall TE, Goetz TG, et al. Transgender data collection in the electronic health record: Current concepts and issues. Journal of the American Medical Informatics Association. 2021:1-14

[4] Ram A, Kronk CA, Eleazer JR, Goulet JL, Brandt CA, Wang KH. Transphobia, encoded: An examination of trans-specific terminology in SNOMED CT and ICD-10-CM. Journal of the American Medical Informatics Association. 2021:1-7

[5] Baldwin A, Dodge B, Schick VR, Light B, Scharrs PW, Herbenick D, et al. Transgender and genderqueer individuals' experiences with healthcare providers: What's working, what's not, and where do we go from here? Journal of Healthcare for the Poor and Underserved. 2018;**29**(4):1300-1318

[6] Kattari SK, Bakko M, Langenderfer-Magruder L, Holloway BT. Transgender and nonbinary experiences of victimization in healthcare. Journal of Interpersonal Violence. 2021;**36**(23-24):NP13054-NP13076. DOI: 10.1177/0886260520905091. Epub 2020 Feb 11

[7] Carrera-Fernández MV, Lameiras-Fernández M, Blanco-Pardo N, Rodríguez-Castro Y. Preventing violence toward sexual and cultural diversity: The role of a queering sex education. International Journal of Environmental Research and Public Health. 2021;**18**(4):2199

[8] Gato J, Leal D, Moleiro C, Fernandes T, Nunes D, Marinho I, et al. "The Worst Part Was Coming Back Home and Feeling Like Crying": Experiences of lesbian, gay, bisexual and trans students in Portuguese schools. Frontiers in Psychology. 2020;**10**:2936

[9] Lau F, Antonio M, Davison K, Queen R, Bryski K. An environmental scan of sex and gender in electronic health records: Analysis of public information sources. Journal of Medical Internet Research. 2020;**22**(11):e20050

[10] Davison K, Queen R, Lau F, Antonio M. Culturally competent gender, sex, and sexual orientation information practices and electronic health records: Rapid review. JMIR Medical Informatics. 2021;**9**(2):e25467

[11] McClure RC, Macumber CL, Kronk C, Grasso C, Horn RJ, Queen R, et al. Gender harmony: Improved standards to support affirmative care of gender-marginalized people through inclusive gender and sex representation. Journal of the American Medical Informatics Association. 2021:1-10

[12] Antonio M, Lau F, Davison K, Devor A, Queen R, Courtney K. Toward an inclusive digital health system for sexual and gender minorities in Canada. Journal of the American Medical Informatics Association. 2021:1-6

[13] Lau F, Antonio M, Davison K, Queen R, Devor A. A rapid review of gender, sex, and sexual orientation documentation in electronic health records. Journal of the American Medical Informatics Association. 2020;**27**(11):1774-1783

[14] Kronk C. Modeling and Operationalizing Gender, Sex and Sexual Orientation: Recommendations and Future Directions [Internet]. Canada Health Infoway Sex-Gender Working Group, University of Cincinatti; 2021 [cited: 2021 Jul 2]. Available from: https://infocentral.infoway-inforoute.ca/en/collaboration/wg/sex-gender

[15] Divan V, Cortez C, Smelyanskaya M, Keatley J. Transgender social inclusion and equality: A pivotal path to development. Journal of the International AIDS Society. 2016;**19**:20803

[16] Swartz TH, Palermo A-GS, Masur SK, Aberg JA. The science and value of diversity: Closing the gaps in our understanding of inclusion and diversity. The Journal of Infectious Diseases. 2019;**220**(Suppl. 2):S33-S41

[17] Rifkin SB. Alma Ata after 40 years: Primary healthcare and health for all—From consensus to complexity. BMJ Global Health. 2018;**3**(Suppl. 3):e001188

[18] Safer JD, Coleman E, Feldman J, Garofalo R, Hembree W, Radix A, et al. Barriers to healthcare for transgender individuals. Current Opinion in Endocrinology, Diabetes, and Obesity. 2016;**23**(2):168-171

[19] Browne AJ, Varcoe C, Ford-Gilboe M, Nadine Wathen C, Smye V, Jackson BE, et al. Disruption as opportunity: Impacts of an organizational health equity intervention in primary care clinics. International Journal for Equity in Health. 2018;**17**(1):154

[20] Kronk C, Tran GQ, Wu DTY. Creating a queer ontology: The gender, sex, and sexual orientation (GSSO) ontology. Studies in Health Technology and Informatics. 2019;**264**:208-212. DOI: 10.3233/SHTI190213

[21] Infoway Sex and Gender Working Group. A Proposed Action Plan to Modernize Gender, Sex and Sexual Orientation Information Practices in Canadian Electronic Health Record Systems. Planning Project [Internet]. Canada Health Infoway; 2021. Available from: https://infocentral.infoway-inforoute.ca/en/resources/docs/3496-gsso-action-plan-full-document/view-document

[22] HL7 International. HL7 Informative Document: Gender Harmony—Modeling Sex and Gender Representation, Release 1 [Internet]. HL7 International; 2021 [cited: 2021 Aug 29]. Available from: https://www.hl7.org/implement/standards/product_brief.cfm?product_id=564

[23] National LGBT Health Education Centre FH. Collecting sexual orientation and gender identity data in electronic health records [Internet]. Fenway Health; 2018. Available from: https://www.lgbtqiahealtheducation.org/wp-content/uploads/Collecting-Sexual-Orientation-and-Gender-Identity-Data-in-EHRs-2016.pdf

[24] Canadian Institute for Health Information. CIHI Reference Data Model Toolkit. p. 105

[25] Office of the National Coordinator for Health Information Technology. United States Core Data for Interoperability Version 2 [Internet]. Office of the National Coordinator for Health Information Technology; 2021 [cited: 2021 Jul 17]. Available from:

https://www.healthit.gov/isa/sites/isa/files/2021-07/USCDI-Version-2-July-2021-Final.pdf

[26] Kluge E-H, Lacroix P, Ruotsalainen P. Ethics certification of health information professionals. Yearbook of Medical Informatics. 2018;**27**(1):037-040

[27] Duggal R, Brindle I, Bagenal J. Digital healthcare: Regulating the revolution. BMJ. 2018;**360**:k6

[28] Taylor L. What is data justice? The case for connecting digital rights and freedoms globally. Big Data & Society. 2017;**4**(2):205395171773633

Chapter 7

Phalloplasty in Transgender Men with and without Urethral Lengthening

Christopher Salgado, Kerstin Yu, Stefan Kenel-Pierre, Edward Gheiler and Tony Shao

Abstract

Our goal in trans man phalloplasty is to decrease the patient's level of gender incongruence, obviate the use of an external prosthesis, be able to orgasm, and give the patient the ability to urinate standing (if desired), while also attempting to decrease urinary complications. The decision to undergo urethral lengthening is considered early in this surgical process. However, urethral complications are among the most common problems we see in phalloplasty, and surgical techniques have evolved to decrease these complications. We have developed an advanced two-stage mucosa-only prelaminated neourethra phalloplasty technique to address these issues. Our surgical technique is detailed in addition to providing patient demographics, co-morbidities, flap complications, and urinary sequelae. We also discuss the perineal urethroplasty in patients opting for no urethral lengthening in phalloplasty. All options should be given and risks considered in trans men undergoing soft tissue phalloplasty, and these will be discussed in detail.

Keywords: phalloplasty, sex reassignment surgery, transition, transgender, urethroplasty

1. Introduction

The radial forearm flap is the most commonly used technique for phalloplasty. The goals of penile construction in a transgender man are to decrease the patient's gender incongruence, obviate the use of an external prosthesis, give the patient the ability to orgasm, and to urinate through the constructed phallus if desired. Urethral strictures and fistulas are common complications following a phalloplasty with urethral lengthening that may be mitigated with a two-stage technique that utilizes a mucosa-only prelaminated neourethra. Sources of the mucosa may include vaginal and oral mucosa and less commonly, uterine, bladder, and colonic mucosa.

Transition of the trans man genitalia is commonly performed in multiple stages including a hysterectomy and oophorectomy primarily and if desired, followed by a vaginectomy with urethral diversion to the perineum or lengthening with a phalloplasty, scrotoplasty, and glansplasty. The ovaries may be preserved at the time of hysterectomy for possible egg preservation. If the decision is made to preserve the ovaries, it is crucial for the patient to be monitored for abnormalities through yearly routine surveillance.

First stage surgery may consist of a hysterectomy and oophorectomy (if not done prior) along with a vaginectomy with urethra lengthening using an anteriorly based vaginal flap with labia minora tissues along with prelamination of the nondominant radial forearm flap using vaginal mucosa, buccal mucosa, and less common skin grafts.

Second stage surgery, which commonly occurs 2–3 months following the first stage, consists of tubularization of the radial forearm tissue with free flap transfer, microvascular anastomosis, neurotization, urethroplasty, scrotoplasty, and glansplasty.

2. Justification for the radial forearm free flap

Given the large cutaneous surface of a native male phallus, autologous construction of a neophallus commonly will necessitate a large cutaneous donor site. Flaps, such as the tube-in-tube radial forearm flap, latissimus dorsi flap, scapular flap, deltoid flap, abdominal pedicled flap, and anterolateral thigh (ALT) flaps have all been used for phalloplasty [1]. Though many techniques have been described, the radial forearm free flap (RFFF) remains the most common for phalloplasty due to its long, reliable vascular pedicle, multiple nerve innervations for anastomosis to the recipient site, and pliability of the tissue facilitating eventual implant placement [2]. In addition, the radial forearm flap has a lower urethral and flap loss complication rate compared to the anterolateral thigh flap [3]. Harvest allows for simultaneous operative sites at the pelvis, upper extremity, and oral region if buccal mucosa is needed. This ability allows for decreased operative time, which can last from 5–12 hours. The RFFF technique makes it possible for patients to fulfill their desires of standing micturition, aesthetic acceptability, and erogenous and tactile sensation.

Erectile rigidity is another commonly reported goal of phalloplasty. To achieve an erection, radial bone can be utilized as an osteocutaneous flap at the time of neophallus creation, or a patient can opt to undergo insertion of a semirigid or hydraulic prosthesis at least 1 year after phalloplasty. It should be noted, however, that our practice prefers to no longer perform the osteocutaneous RFFF due to dyspareunia experienced by the patient post-surgery. This is due to the anchoring of the radius bone at the pubic symphysis. Additionally, most centers report a 30%+ extrusion rate necessitating implant removal at 2–3 years, and reoperation rates reach 100% at 5 years (**Figure 1**) [4]. There is a significant risk of complications following placement of penile prosthesis including mechanical failure, infection, and mal-positioning. It is critical to have a plastic surgeon trained in microvascular surgery present during the placement of the penile implant as the vascular pedicle may be readily injured during the dissection and subsequent dilation process required for placement of the cylinders. It is critical to avoid multiple passing of the dilators so that devascularization of the phallus does not ensue.

Adding to the complexity of phalloplasty is the creation of a functional penile urethra. The urethra after neophallus construction can be divided into distinct segments, from proximal to distal: native (female) urethra, fixed or lengthened urethra, the anastomotic urethra, penile shaft urethra, and external meatus. The fixed urethra is the portion of the urethra formed after lengthening the native urethra via local vaginal or labial flaps, extragenital flaps, and grafts of skin or mucosa (**Figure 2**). The phallic urethra can be constructed by prelamination, tube-in-tube techniques, or pedicle flaps [2].

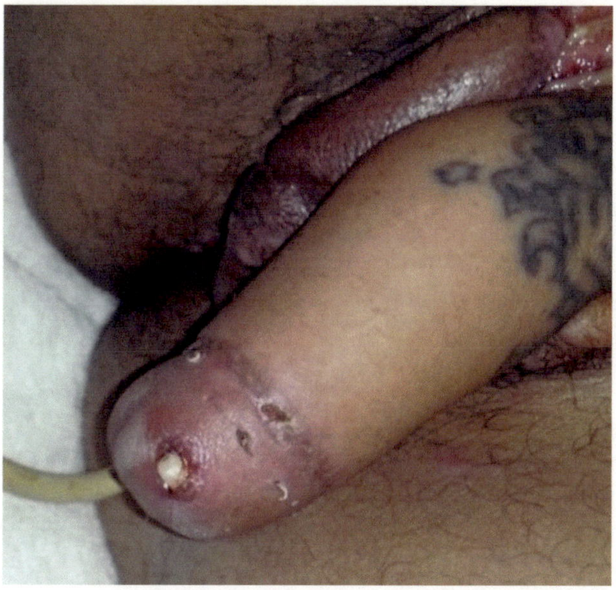

Figure 1.
Radius bone exposure following radial forearm osteocutaneous flap phalloplasty.

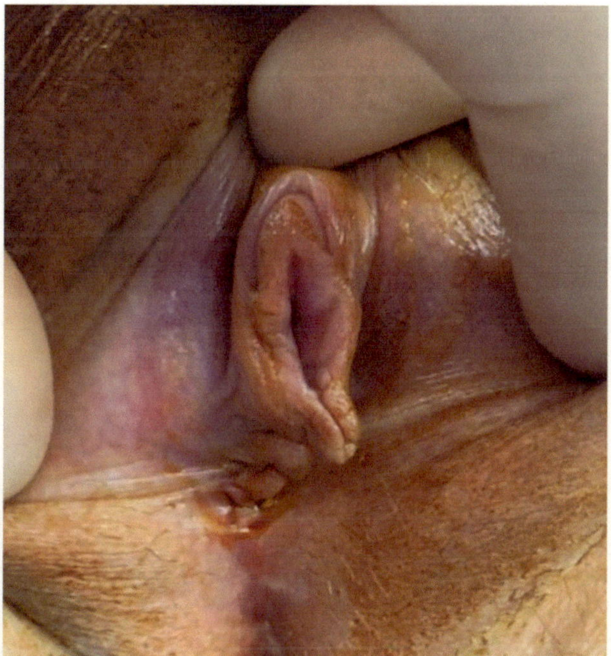

Figure 2.
Patient 3 months following urethral lengthening using labia minora and anterior vaginal wall flaps.

2.1 Inflow for phalloplasty: preoperative assessment

The preoperative assessment begins with a physical examination. The patient is assessed for adequate perfusion to the lower extremities. Ideally, the patient should have a palpable pedal pulse bilaterally. If perfusion is in question especially when dealing with patients with peripheral arterial disease, one can obtain noninvasive studies such as arterial duplex or plethysmography to determine which side to use. Preoperative vein mapping can be performed to assess for deep venous thrombosis as well as the caliber and quality of the great saphenous vein. Ideally, the great saphenous vein should be 2.5–3 mm and free of sclerosis.

2.2 Branch of profunda femoris artery

A branch of the profunda femoris artery is an option for inflow. The perfusion to the thigh is robust thus a branch of the profunda femoris artery can typically be sacrificed without significantly affecting thigh perfusion. To expose the profunda femoris artery, a longitudinal skin incision is made in the thigh overlying the femoral arteries. The femoral bifurcation is identified and the superficial femoral artery is preserved. The main trunk of the profunda femoris artery is identified and preserved. There are tributary branches of the profunda femoris vein that are ligated to facilitate exposure and hemostasis. The branches of the profunda femoris artery are identified and circumferentially dissected. Typically, the ascending branch is of adequate caliber and length to be used for the inflow. If this branch is not long enough or the caliber is too small, the remaining branches of the profunda can be explored.

2.3 Great saphenous vein to femoral artery transposition in a loop configuration (loop graft)

An alternative source of inflow can be the superficial femoral artery or the common femoral artery. The great saphenous vein can be used as a conduit. An oblique incision is made in the medial groin overlying the femoral artery bifurcation as well as the saphenofemoral junction. The saphenous vein is identified first and preserved. The superficial femoral artery is then exposed that lies medial to the femoral vein. The artery is sequentially dissected and controlled, and the skin incision is extended distally along the course of the saphenous vein. The length of the vein needed to perform the loop transposition varies by patient. The length required can be estimated with a free tie. Ideally, the loop graft needs to be able to reach the pubis when is oriented medially. Once the saphenous vein is exposed, it is circumferentially dissected and its tributary branches are ligated and divided. Careful attention needs to be made when ligating the branches too close to the vein as it may cause stenosis. The saphenous vein is then transected distally, and the distal end is ligated. The vein is then cannulated and distended with heparinized saline solution. Any defects are identified and repaired. When the vein is distended, it is marked for orientation. To perform the loop configuration, the distal end of the vein is swung in a counterclockwise fashion toward the femoral artery. The patient is systemically heparinized. The femoral artery was clamped proximally and distally and an arteriotomy is made using 11 blades and then lengthened with Potts scissors. Alternatively, an aortic punch device can be used to enlarge the arteriotomy to the desired size. The anastomosis should be approximately 4 mm. An end-to-side anastomosis was performed between the femoral artery and the saphenous vein paying careful attention to maintaining the orientation of the vein to avoid twisting and kinking. Just prior to completing the last few sutures of the anastomosis, the femoral artery is forward and back-bled. The lumen of the artery and vein are flushed with heparinized saline solution to flush any thrombus. Once the anastomosis is completed, the clamps are released. The loop graft is assessed for orientation and flow. The patient's leg and foot also need to be assessed to ensure there are no changes to baseline perfusion. One can expect a weak pulse and a thrill when palpating the graft. A Doppler can also be used to assess the presence of flow. If the loop graft is kinked or twisted, it may thrombose. When the loop graft is ready to be used, it is transected in the middle; the proximal end is the arterial inflow and the distal end is the venous outflow.

2.4 Complications of urinary stricture and fistula

Complications of urinary stricture and fistula are prevalent. Variations of urethral lengthening techniques among centers have resulted from attempts to improve upon urologic complication rates, which range from 33 to 77% in large case series [5]. Urethral cutaneous fistulas following surgery may range from 22 to 75% [6]. Fistulas occur most commonly at or just proximal to the anastomosis between the phallic urethra and fixed urethra due to vascular insufficiency of the flap and decreased lumen of the phallic urethra. Rates of urethral strictures in female-to-male phalloplasty recipients range from 11 to 74% [7–9]. Since the plastic surgeon alone is not trained in the management of urethral strictures or fistulas, we believe it is essential to have a qualified reconstructive urologist involved in the management of these complications to optimize patient care.

The radial forearm flap may allow the patient to have penetrative sexual intercourse, has minimal donor site scarring, results in a cosmetically acceptable phallus, has tactile and erogenous sensitivity, and potentially creates a competent neourethra that allows for standing urination. These ideal characteristics, described by Hage et al, are mostly met by the RFFF (radial forearm free flap) [10].

Recognizing that urethral strictures and fistulas remain the most challenging complication we face, we have been able to decrease their occurrence with a staged technique. We have found that the radial forearm tube-within-a-tube technique not only requires electrolysis of the forearm to avoid hair growth within the urethra—a common cause of stricture—but also requires a larger donor site since flap skin is used to create the urethra. Minimizing the donor site and decreasing stricture rates

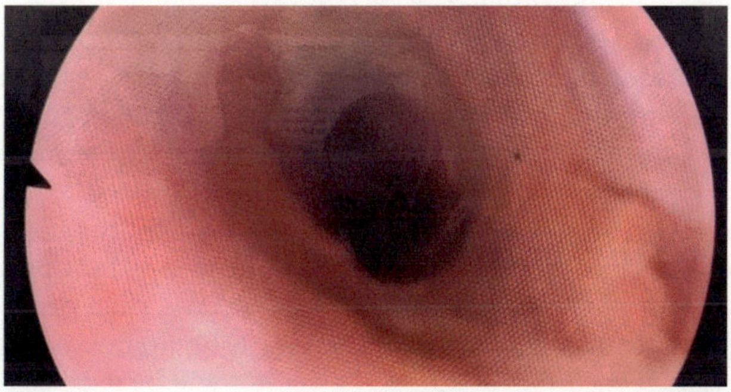

Figure 3.
Cystoscopy of prelaminated neourethra prior to stage 2 phalloplasty revealing mucosa which mimics that of native urethral mucosa.

have encouraged us to continue the two-stage technique with mucosal prelamination, which more closely mimics native urethra mucosa (**Figure 3**).

3. Patient evaluation

Given the potential morbidity associated with the complex phalloplasty procedure, an adequate preoperative evaluation is essential. The need for gender dysphoria evaluation and medical clearance is unique to this patient population. Gender identity disorder or gender incongruence is classified by the International Classification of Disease Manual as ICD-10-CM F64.9. The DSM-5 defines gender dysphoria as an incongruity between the patient's experienced and expressed gender and their assigned gender, which causes clinically significant distress lasting at least 6 months, however, this has often lasted nearly the individual's entire life [11]. According to the World Professional Association for Transgender Health (WPATH), a psychological evaluation and two letters recommending gender affirmation surgery from two psychiatrists or licensed mental health therapists, who independently assessed the patient, are required for the removal of reproductive organs and/or phalloplasty [12]. In addition, the patient must have taken hormone replacement therapy and lived as their true gender for at least 1 year. These prerequisites are not only required by most insurance companies for authorization of the procedure but also ensure that patients have a realistic understanding of the procedure and serve to minimize disappointment and patient regret.

The importance of a thorough preoperative psychosocial evaluation cannot be overstated. Adequate social support is encouraged to facilitate a successful recovery. The patient should be informed to expect frequent postoperative visits 1–2 months following surgery and should understand that the operation will impact their ability to work for 4–6 weeks. The surgeon should remain involved in all stages of the preoperative evaluation by corresponding with the patient's mental health provider and urogynecologist.

A clear and candid discussion regarding the patient's desired goals from surgery, including the length and circumference of the neophallus, allows the surgeon to determine whether expectations are realistic given the patient's anatomy. The limitations, functional outcomes, recovery, risk of complications, timing of procedures, and cost of each surgery should be honestly discussed with the patient.

It is critical to accurately document current medications, including antiplatelet agents and hormones, in addition to the patient's smoking history. Androgens such as testosterone must be discontinued 2 weeks prior to surgery to reduce the risk of thrombosis, and smoking cessation is required 4 weeks prior to surgery and up to 4 weeks after to ensure proper healing. Specific information regarding prior infections helps in selecting postoperative antibiotics, as postsurgical infection will delay healing and increase morbidity.

The microsurgical component of RFFF phalloplasty requires additional preoperative evaluation. Adequate recipient vessels will be needed for the microsurgical construction. If arterial inflow from the thigh will be used then pedal vessels should be assessed for adequate inflow. The abdominal wall should be examined for prior incisions particularly if the inferior epigastric vessels will be used as recipient's vessels. We have used the inferior epigastric artery, descending branch of the lateral femoral circumflex or on occasion arterio-venous loops for recipient arteries and the inferior epigastric vein or saphenous veins for recipient venous outflow.

Allen's test of the patient's nondominant hand confirms that harvest of the RFFF flap will not compromise the blood supply to the hand. If the results of Allen's test are poor, that is, the hand remains cool and pale after the release of ulnar artery occlusion, using another donor site should be considered or the dominant forearm. In addition, sensitive tattoos of the proposed forearm should be evaluated. Patients who live in cold climates may need reconstitution of their arterial anatomy with vein grafts after flap harvest.

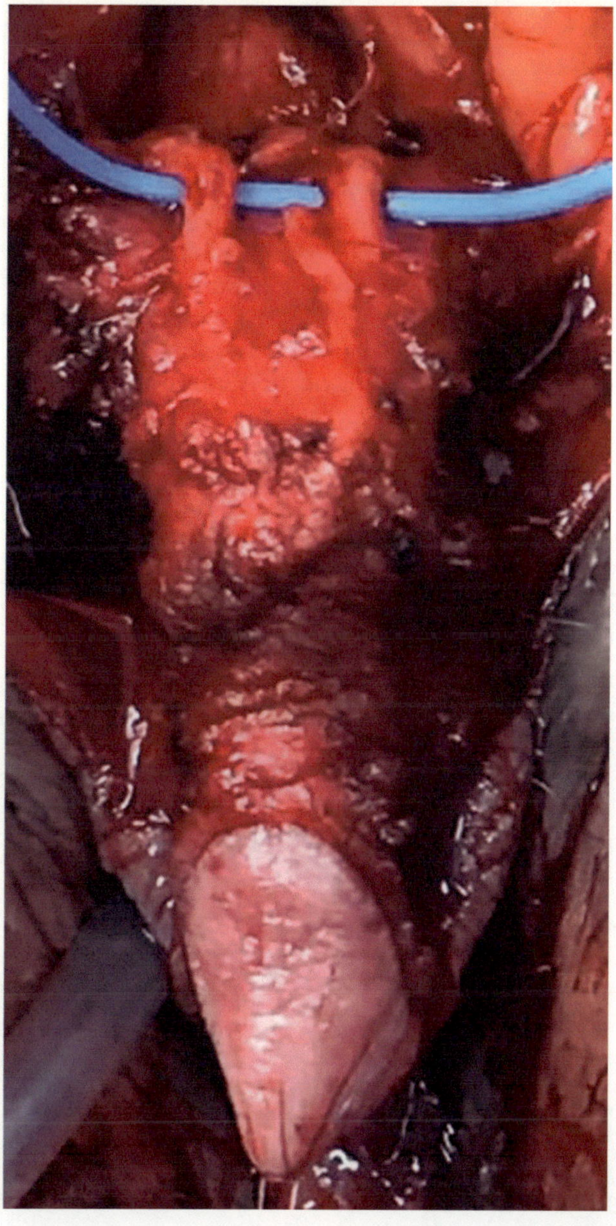

Figure 4.
Clitoral nerves are exposed as recipient's nerves at stage 2 RFFF phalloplasty.

Prior to surgery, it is also vital to assess patient sensation to determine if orgasm can be achieved through clitoral stimulation. The dorsal clitoral nerve (**Figure 4**), ilioinguinal nerve, and genitofemoral nerve co-apted to the medial and lateral antebrachial cutaneous nerves will provide both erogenous and protective sensation to the neophallus. If a patient has difficulty achieving orgasm prior to surgery, it is unlikely that the patient will be able to after surgery.

It should also be noted that part of the patient population has forearm tattoos that will affect the cosmesis of the neophallus. Patient preference will dictate whether the presence of forearm tattoos on the neophallus is acceptable. Clear expectations should be set with the patient regarding the forearm donor site scar, which may be perceived as a stigma, however, we argue the scar is more acceptable than the anterolateral thigh flap scar (**Figure 5**).

3.1 Preoperative preparation

In our practice, we construct the penile urethra by forearm prelamination with mucosa, which obviates the need for forearm depilation (as would be the case in a tube-within-a-tube technique). The native urethra is a fibromuscular tube lined by urothelium, columnar epithelium, and nonkeratinizing squamous epithelium. Mucosal grafts have greater homology to the native urethra as they are also composed of nonkeratinized epithelium, which has led to less scar contracture and subsequent urethral strictures and fistulas following neourethral construction [1].

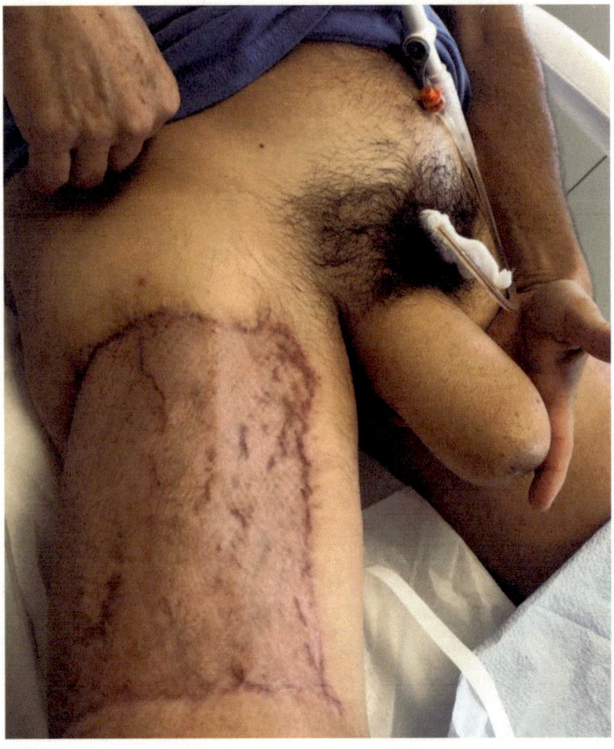

Figure 5.
Patient with urethral and flap-related complications following ALT phalloplasty from an outlying institution.

Prior to phalloplasty, a patient should have had a hysterectomy and oophorectomy. If he has not yet had these procedures, it is possible to have them performed during the first stage of our approach to staged phalloplasty. We have found that uterine mucosa is readily available if the patient is undergoing hysterectomy in the same operative setting as phalloplasty, and can be used to construct a patent, functional penile urethra [1]. If a patient is interested in egg harvesting prior to oophorectomy, this is performed before definitive and irreversible hysterectomy and oophorectomy.

The current sequence of surgery in our practice is first a subcutaneous mastectomy, followed by a hysterectomy and oophorectomy combined with a vaginectomy, scrotoplasty, and reconstruction of the horizontal part of the urethra, and later the actual phalloplasty.

3.2 Surgical technique

We have found our two-stage technique allows for a urethral conduit which mimics that of a native urethra with no hair growth while minimizing the donor site on the forearm. Our decreased stricture rate has encouraged us to continue the use of this technique in patients pursuing phalloplasty with urethral lengthening.

3.3 Stage 1: prelamination technique

The main procedures are as follows:

1. Vaginectomy with the harvest of vaginal mucosa tissue (combined with hysterectomy and oophorectomy if not already performed)—Procedure performed concurrently by urogynecologist or gynecologic oncologist

2. Urethral lengthening utilizing labia minora flaps and anteriorly based vaginal mucosa flap harvested at the time of vaginectomy

3. Occasional harvest of buccal mucosa if required for neo-urethra

4. Radial forearm flap elevation ulnarly for flap urethra prelamination

IV antibiotics against gram-positive, gram-negative organisms and anaerobes are administered to the patient 1 hour prior to incision.

The first stage entails flap prelamination during which the radial forearm flap is designed and the neourethra is formed using autologous tissue; mucosa is preferentially used in our practice. The markings for the planned flap are determined preoperatively following a normal Allen's test on the patient's nondominant upper extremity, ensuring that the patient's hand can be perfused with the ulnar artery alone. The flap is elevated from the ulnar to radial direction in the supra-fascial plane to allow placement of the neourethra.

Prelamination of the patient's eventual penile urethra is performed by grafting vaginal, and/or buccal mucosa in a suprafascial plane of the donor volar and ulnar forearm. The vaginal mucosa is harvested during the vaginectomy for the creation of the neourethra. We lengthen the native female urethra using labia minora tissues and an anterior pedicled vaginal flap. If a hysterectomy has not already been performed, it can be performed during this stage to provide additional mucosal tissue for the neourethra. The buccal mucosa is also harvested at this time if necessary (**Figures 6** and 7). To allow

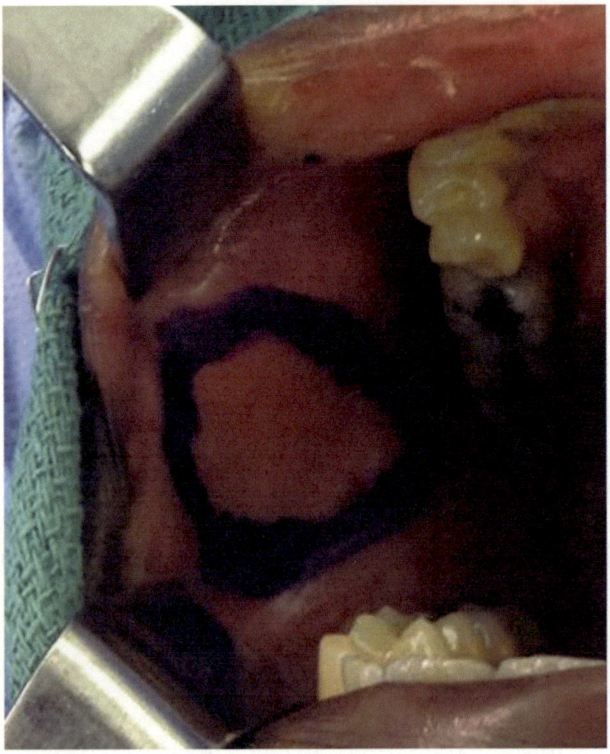

Figure 6.
Markings of buccal mucosal graft. Avoid injury to Stenson's duct.

for irrigation of the entire prelaminated neourethra, holes are cut into a 24-French Foley. After mucosal harvest, the mucosal grafts are cleansed with a betadine and normal saline solution and then sewed around the holed catheter construct, exteriorizing the sub-mucosal surface using a running, locking suture. Placing this construct lengthwise in the subcutaneous forearm (suprafascial plane) allows for the creation of a tubular graft, which will become the penile neourethra of the eventual phalloplasty. The patient is then immobilized in a splint for several days. Irrigation of the prelaminated flap is then performed twice daily beginning 1 week after surgery, a practice continued until flap transfer to prevent infection.

Creating the urethra with mucosal tissue and not using forearm tissue decreases the width of the flap skin paddle compared to the traditional tube-within-a-tube urethra and yields a more aesthetically acceptable donor site scar. With this method, the patient can place his upper extremity across his chest with the flexor aspect against the chest and the scar will not be visible (**Figure 8**). Furthermore, with this technique, the patient does not need to undergo costly depilation treatments as there will be no hair growth within the urethra. Prelamination can also be completed with a skin graft from the thigh or abdomen when mucosal tissue is inadequate in patients who have undergone metoidioplasty with vaginectomy, however, this may lead to increased stricture rates.

3.4 Stage 2: radial forearm free flap transfer

Approximately 8–12 weeks after the first stage flap prelamination, creation of the neophallus can be performed. Although allowing more time between stages may be

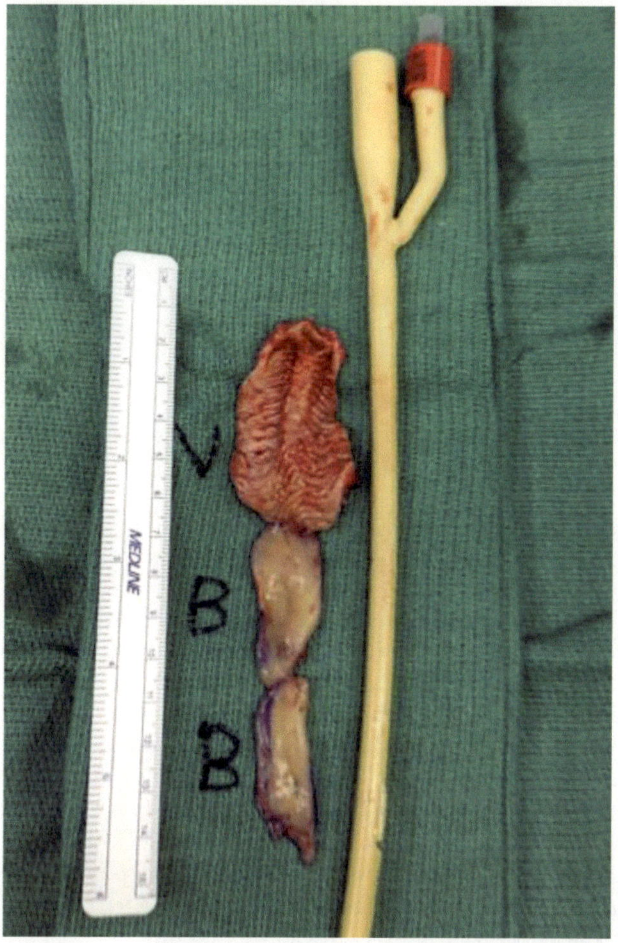

Figure 7.
Vaginal and buccal mucosa with mucosal surface toward the foley catheter in preparation for tubularization around the catheter.

favorable, we have found that 8 weeks is long enough to achieve successful wound healing and favorable results and is a time frame that is tolerable for our patients [1].

One hour before incision is made, antibiotics against gram-positive, gram-negative, and anaerobic organisms should be intravenously administered to the patient. A tourniquet is used for flap harvest, in addition to a hand table. Separate surgical set-ups are used for the pelvic area and upper extremity to avoid cross-contamination. Two surgical teams can work simultaneously—one team performs the RFFF harvest and the second team performs the dissection of the recipient's vessels (inferior epigastric artery and vein and/or descending branch of the lateral circumflex artery and saphenous vein), recipient nerves, preparation of the urethra for anastomosis and scrotoplasty.

The design of the radial forearm flap was defined in the first stage. A marking pen is used to delineate the dimensions of the flap, which will commonly measure 5.5–7.5 inches in length and 5.5–6.5 inches in width. Whereas the flap was elevated in the suprafascial plane for prelamination at Stage I, the flap is now elevated in the subfascial plane to avoid injury to the neourethra. The dissection begins on the ulnar side of

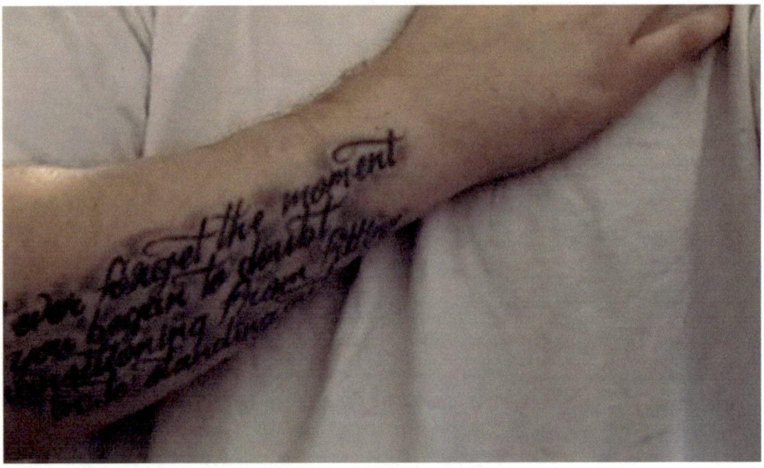

Figure 8.
Patient following staged radial forearm flap harvest revealing limited donor site secondary due to prelamination of the urethra.

the forearm and proceeds to the flexor carpi radialis and brachioradialis tendons for the RFFF harvest. The medial and lateral antebrachial cutaneous nerves are preserved during dissection of the radial forearm flap for coaptation to one dorsal nerve of the clitoris end-to-side for erogenous sensation and the ilioinguinal or genitofemoral nerve for tactile sensation. The radial artery and venae comitantes are ligated distally and proximally dissected for vascular anastomosis. Prior to distal ligation, the artery may be temporarily clamped to ensure blood flow to the hand. The basilic and/or cephalic veins are preserved and dissected with the flap. While the RFFF remains connected to its inherent blood supply, the flap is tubed into a phallus and sutured so that the neourethra is buried within the tubed phallus (**Figure 9**).

Using a modification of Monstrey's scrotoplasty technique, the clitoris is dissected free from the lengthened urethra and denuded of skin [13]. The clitoral hood skin is removed and used for the coronaplasty using a technique described by Gottlieb [14] (**Figure 10**). The recipient arteries harvested for the vascular anastomoses are either the inferior epigastric artery or the descending branch of the lateral femoral circumflex

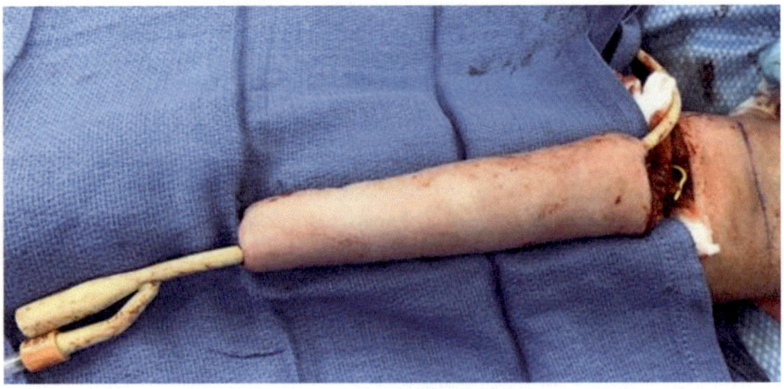

Figure 9.
Tubed radial forearm flap at the donor site with the prelaminated urethra.

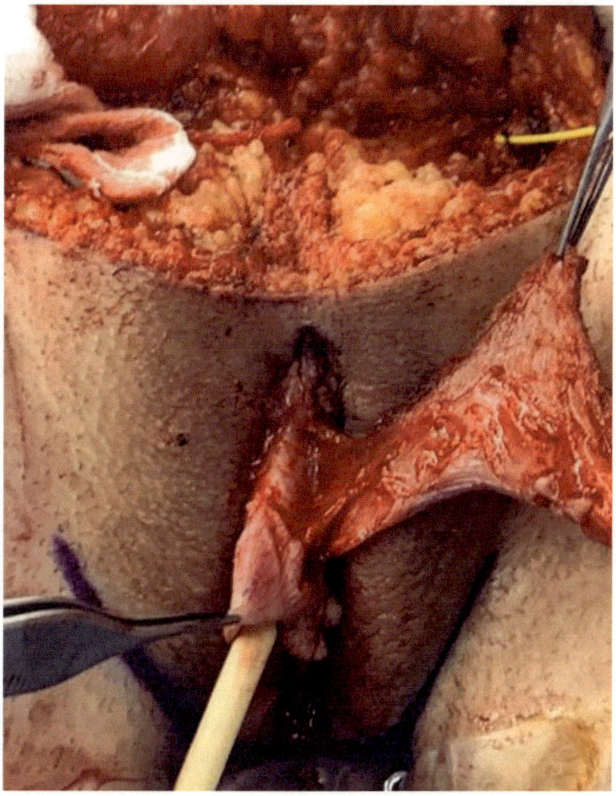

Figure 10.
Trans male patient during the harvest of clitoral (or T-dick) hood skin for coronaplasty using Gottlieb technique.

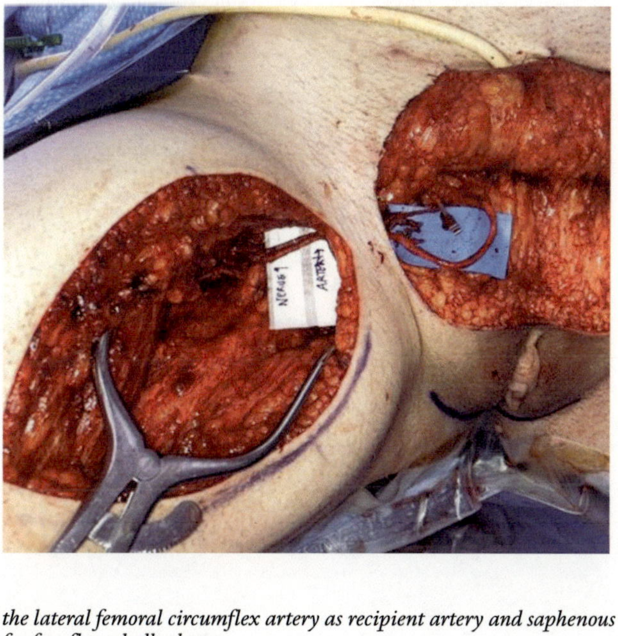

Figure 11.
Descending branch of the lateral femoral circumflex artery as recipient artery and saphenous vein as recipient artery in preparation for free flap phalloplasty.

artery. Of note, once we switched to using the descending branch of the lateral femoral circumflex artery as our recipient artery, we no longer had re-open procedures due to vascular compromise [2]. The thigh incision made for the lateral femoral circumflex is also used for the harvest of the great saphenous vein (**Figure 11**). Since we use the greater saphenous veins as recipient veins for the radial forearm flap, the proximal incision made to harvest the greater saphenous vein is also used for the gracilis muscle harvest. The distal free end of the muscle, harvested via a separate distal incision, is delivered through the proximal incision. Undermining of the soft tissues is performed from the proximal thigh incision to the level of the midline groin defect where the urethral anastomosis is to be performed.

After vessel preparation with a microscope and confirming adequate outflow from the descending branch of the lateral femoral circumflex artery and inflow from the great saphenous vein, the RFFF is transferred to the pubic area. The forearm donor site can be covered with either an autologous split-thickness skin graft or the surgeon can apply a dermal substitute that can be grafted later. The first maneuver is to place the foley catheter, which is located in the neourethra, directly into the patient's bladder. Absorbable sutures are used for the urethral anastomosis in two layers, which is the first anastomosis performed (**Figure 12**).

The arterial, venous, and neural anastomoses are performed next in that order and are all hand-sewn using 9-0 nylon suture with the aid of an operative microscope. The radial artery is connected end-to-end to the descending branch of the lateral circumflex artery. The venous anastomosis is performed between the cephalic or basilic vein and the greater saphenous vein. A second venous anastomosis can be performed between a radial venous comitante vein with the contralateral greater saphenous vein. Two to three nerve anastomoses may also be performed. The medial and lateral antebrachial cutaneous nerves are anastomosed end-to-end to the ilioinguinal nerves

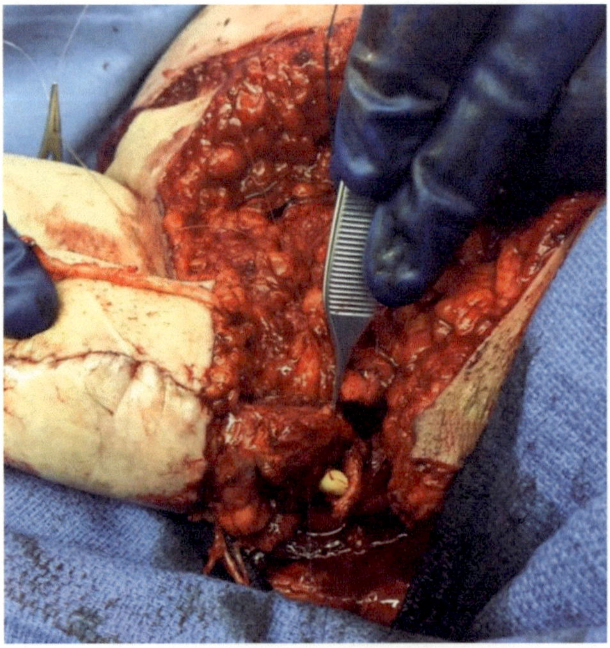

Figure 12.
First of two-layered urethral anastomosis in staged radial forearm flap phalloplasty.

and to one of the dorsal clitoral nerves end-to-side. The ilioinguinal nerve is commonly found exiting the external inguinal ring. A cadaver nerve graft may be used as an interposition nerve graft when needed.

The gracilis muscle may be harvested in a minimally invasive fashion and wrapped around the urethral anastomosis, avoiding compression of the vascular pedicle, to provide vascularity to a minimally vascular urethral anastomosis (**Figure 13**). This maneuver also provides bulk to the neo-scrotum often obviating the need for scrotal implants. At our institution, we have been able to minimize urethral fistula rates using a gracliis muscle flap to augment the urethral anastomosis [15].

A suprapubic tube is placed and used for urinary diversion if needed during urinary training of the neo-phallus.

Upon closure of all incisions, a Norfolk coronaplasty is performed with either a skin graft or labial graft obtained from the clitoral hood region by denuding the clitoris before transposition (**Figure 10**) [16].

Following surgery, patients are transferred to the intensive care unit for flap monitoring and will remain on strict bed rest for a minimum of 3 days. An implantable Doppler device has been very helpful in flap monitoring. Prophylaxis for microvascular thrombosis is typically subcutaneous heparin and aspirin. Strict monitoring of the free tissue transfer is performed by the intensive care unit and resident staff [17]. Patients whose forearm donor site was first covered with a dermal substitute are taken back to the operating room for definitive coverage with a skin graft after 2 weeks. Several days later the patient may be discharged home with both a penile catheter and suprapubic catheter (**Figure 14**). A pericatheter retrograde cystourethrogram can be planned 12 weeks post-surgery. If there is no extravasation of dye, indicating that there is no urinary fistula, the foley catheter can be removed and the suprapubic catheter can be clamped (**Figure 15**). Patients are encouraged to urinate through their neophallus with the suprapubic catheter clamped. We then check for residual urine in the bladder using a bladder scan if necessary. If the patient is successfully able to urinate from the phallus and adequately empty the bladder for several days the suprapubic tube can be discontinued.

If the patient desires, he can tattoo the glans and shaft of the neophallus for aesthetic enhancement, which is ideally performed before full tactile sensation has been achieved

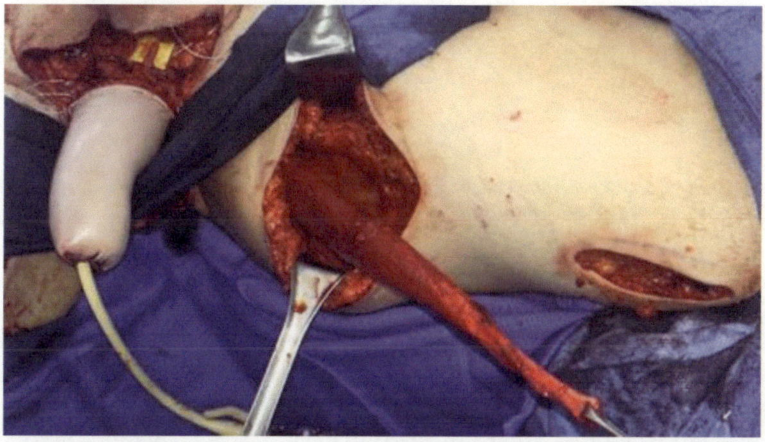

Figure 13.
Gracilis muscle harvest via minimally invasive approach prior to alpha wrap around the urethral anastomosis.

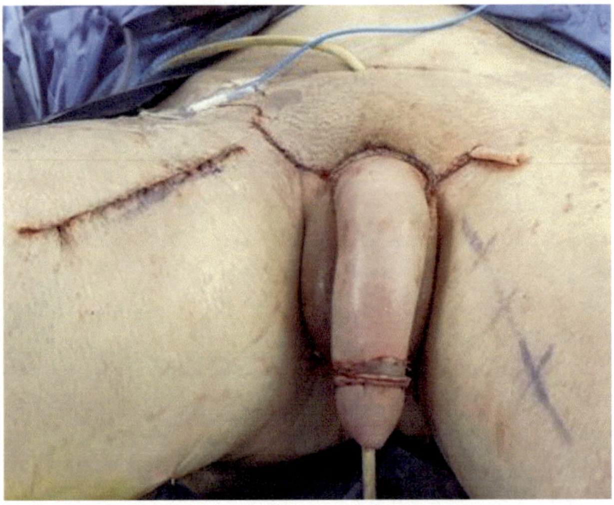

Figure 14.
Trans man following Stage II phalloplasty revealing suprapubic tube and penile foley catheter.

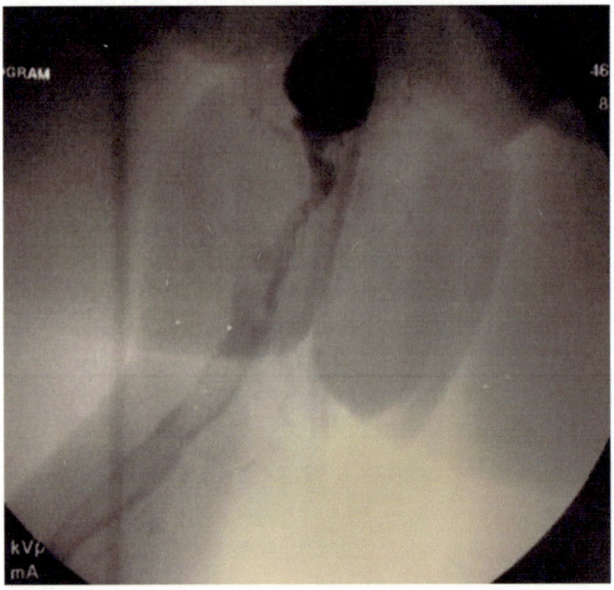

Figure 15.
Pericatheter retrograde cystourethrogram 8 weeks following second stage phalloplasty operation in trans man. The study reveals no contrast extravasation indicating no fistula and no stricture noted.

(typically 1-year postop). Similarly, the donor site can be tattooed to avoid the stigmata of a skin graft (**Figure 16**).

Since the RFFF phalloplasty lacks bone, it may be too soft to allow for penetrative intercourse. Implantation of an erectile prosthesis is a definitive procedure, that may be performed after 8–12 months when tactile sensation is achieved at least ¾ distally of the penile shaft. A simple Tinel sign is often used to assess postoperative tactile sensation in the neo-phallus postoperatively. Both malleable dual or single cylinder

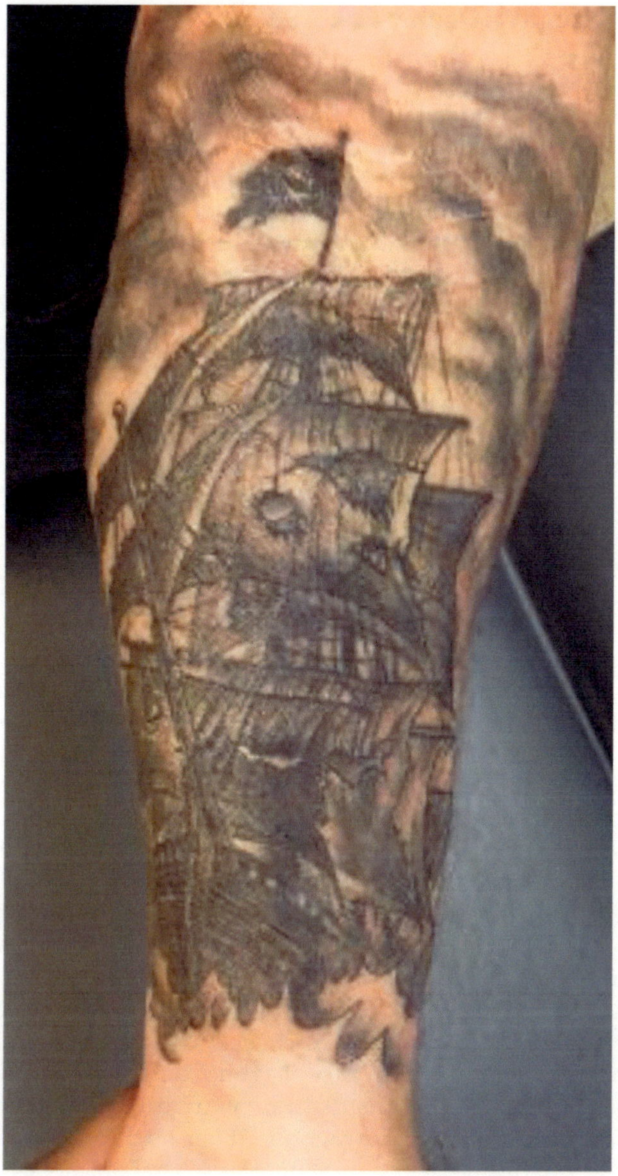

Figure 16.
RFFF donor site with tattoo concealment.

penile prostheses or inflatable prostheses may be used for the erectile device commonly anchored to the ischial tuberosities. We strongly recommend plastic surgery involvement in placement of the prosthesis since knowledge of the location and preservation of the neo-phallus vascular supply is critical to successful placement. More technical details of the neo-phallus implant placement will be discussed in a separate chapter. Prior to implant placement, as the patient is awaiting neural sensation, patients may have successful penetrative intercourse by using an elastic 3M Coban wrap and a condom.

4. Postoperative sequelae/complications

It is important that the patient is aware of the potential complications that may occur following surgery, included in the informed consent. Some complications may include partial or total flap loss, hematoma at the donor or recipient site, an insensate flap, anorgasmia, skin graft loss, chronic pain, numbness, urinary complications, hypertrophic scarring, infection, cold intolerance, vascular compromise, abdominal wall weakness or hernia, implant infection or malfunction, dyspareunia, tendon exposure, limited hand function, and persistent gender dysphoria.

Urethral fistulas and strictures are common untoward events following phalloplasty in the transgender male and may prevent the patient from voiding while standing. A meta-analysis of 665 patients drawn from 11 studies found that an average of 0.51 strictures and/or fistulas can be expected per free forearm flap phalloplasty [17]. The published rate of urologic complications following penile reconstruction ranges from 23 to 75% [18, 19]. The subsequent management of urethral fistulas and strictures can be challenging. Initially, conservative measures such as periodic urethral dilatation or internal urethrotomy can be employed as temporizing measures prior to definitive surgical management.

Most urethral fistulas occur at the anastomosis between the fixed urethra and phallic urethra, and often can occur proximal to a concomitant stricture. The techniques for fistula repair described are the simple fistula repair, the use of local tissue transfer, two-stage procedures with use of mesh graft, bladder, or buccal mucosa [20]. When the fistula is small with substantial overlying tissue, spontaneous resolution is likely. However, when a urethrocutaneous fistula is large and superficial, the above-mentioned surgical repair is necessary.

Urethral strictures also primarily occur at the anastomotic urethra. The keystone surgical procedures for urethral stricture include urethroplasty (excision and primary anastomosis) and staged Johanson-type urethroplasty with additional skin grafts, preferentially buccal mucosa [21]. Surgical approaches are customized to the length of the stricture. A patient who has both a urethral fistula and stricture should have both problems addressed at the same time.

There are many variations of urethroplasty available owing to the considerable heterogeneity of phallic and neourethral construction techniques. Well-vascularized local flaps are utilized when available, as well as buccal mucosal grafts. A patient who has undergone several urethral fistula and/or stricture repair attempts will have progressively fewer options for reconstruction. At our institution, we have significantly decreased our fistula rates in transgender male phalloplasty by augmenting the paucity of vascularized tissue at this anastomosis using a pedicled gracilis flap at the time of flap transfer [15]. Prelamination with mucosal grafts may also decrease urethral stenosis and fistula formation [2].

5. Conclusion

The goals of phalloplasty include a sensate, cosmetically acceptable phallus with an incorporated neourethra, and the ability to place an implantable penile prosthesis to allow rigidity for penetrative intercourse. In the majority of cases, phalloplasty is the final stage of treatment for gender dysphoria.

While other donor sites may be used, the radial forearm free flap is a favorable technique due to its high vascularity, adequate sensation, sufficient tissue pliability, and good cosmetic outcome. We have found that our two-stage technique allows for a neourethra, which mimics a native urethra with no hair growth, while minimizing the donor site on the forearm compared to the previously used skin for a tube-within-a-tube radial forearm flap technique. Using a pre-laminated urethra our patients do not need to undergo electrolysis since the urethra is not created from forearm tissue, so we do not have the risk of hair growth in the urethra and its associated complications. Our decreased stricture rate has encouraged us to continue the use of this technique in patients pursuing phalloplasty with urethral lengthening. Although there have not been any blinded, randomized controlled trials comparing single-stage to two-stage phalloplasty, we believe that prelamination using mucosa for the construction of the trans male phallus urethra is a worthwhile technique that has demonstrated a reduction in the prevalence of complications with this already very challenging procedure.

Conflict of interest

The authors declare no conflict of interest.

Author details

Christopher Salgado[1*], Kerstin Yu[1], Stefan Kenel-Pierre[1], Edward Gheiler[1] and Tony Shao[2]

1 Constructive Surgery Associates, Miami, FL, USA

2 Division of Vascular and Endovascular Surgery, University of Miami, Miami, FL, USA

*Address all correspondence to: miamiplasticsurgeon@hotmail.com

References

[1] Salgado CJ, Fein LA, Chim J, Medina CA, Demaso S, Gomez C. Prelamination of neourethra with uterine mucosa in radial forearm osteocutaneous free flap phalloplasty in the female-to-male transgender patient. Case Reports in Urology. 2016;**2016**:8742531. DOI: 10.1155/2016/8742531. [Epub: 16 Mar 2016].

[2] Salgado CJ, Nugent A, Hadeed J, Lalama M, Rey J, Medina C. Two-stage prelaminated mucosal neourethra radial forearm flap phalloplasty for transgender men. Global Journal of Medical Research. 2021;**1**(1):1-13

[3] Xu KY, Watt AJ. The pedicled anterolateral thigh phalloplasty. Clinics in Plastic Surgery. 2018;**45**(3):399-406

[4] Hoebeke PB, Decaestecker K, Beysens M, Opdenakker Y, Lumen N, Monstrey SM. Erectile implants in female-to-male transsexuals: Our experience in 129 patients. European Urology. 2010;**57**(2):334-341

[5] Monstrey S, Hoebeke P, Selvaggi G, Ceulemans P, Van Landuyt K, Blondeel P, et al. Penile reconstruction: Is the radial forearm flap really the standard technique? Plastic and Reconstructive Surgery. 2009;**124**(2):510-518

[6] Al-Tamimi M, Pigot GL, van der Sluis WB, van de Grift TC, Mullender MG, Groenman F, et al. Colpectomy significantly reduces the risk of urethral fistula formation after urethral lengthening in transgender men undergoing genital gender affirming surgery. The Journal of Urology. 2018;**200**(6):1315-1322

[7] Rohrmann D, Jakse G. Urethroplasty in female-to-male transsexuals. European Urology. 2003;**44**(5):611-614

[8] Leriche A, Timsit MO, Morel-Journel N, Bouillot A, Dembele D, Ruffion A. Long-term outcome of forearm flee-flap phalloplasty in the treatment of transsexualism. BJU International. 2008;**101**(10):1297-1300

[9] Kim SK, Moon JB, Heo J, Kwon YS, Lee KC. A new method of urethroplasty for prevention of fistula in female-to-male gender reassignment surgery. Annals of Plastic Surgery. 2010;**64**(6):759-764

[10] Joris Hage J, De Graaf FH. Addressing the ideal requirements by free flap phalloplasty: Some reflections on refinements of technique. Microsurgery. 1993;**14**(9):592-598

[11] Edition F. Diagnostic and statistical manual of mental disorders. American Psychiatric Association. 2013;**21**:591-643

[12] Coleman E, Bockting W, Botzer M, Cohen-Kettenis P, DeCuypere G, Feldman J, et al. Standards of care for the health of transsexual, transgender, and gender-nonconforming people, version 7. International Journal of Transgenderism. 2012;**13**(4):165-232

[13] Selvaggi G, Hoebeke P, Ceulemans P, Hamdi M, Van Landuyt K, Blondeel P, et al. Scrotal reconstruction in female-to-male transsexuals: A novel scrotoplasty. Plastic and Reconstructive Surgery. 2009;**123**(6):1710-1718

[14] Gottlieb LJ, Levine LA. A new design for the radial forearm free-flap phallic construction. Plastic and Reconstructive Surgery. 1993;**92**(2):276-283

[15] Salgado CJ, Nugent AG, Moody AM, Chim H, Paz AM, Chen HC. Immediate pedicled gracilis flap in radial forearm flap phalloplasty for transgender male

patients to reduce urinary fistula. Journal of Plastic, Reconstructive & Aesthetic Surgery. 2016;**69**(11):1551-1557

[16] Gilbert DA, Jordan GH, Devine CJ Jr, Winslow BH. Microsurgical forearm "cricket bat-transformer" phalloplasty. Plastic and Reconstructive Surgery. 1992;**90**(4):711-716

[17] Frey JD, Poudrier G, Chiodo MV, Hazen A. A systematic review of metoidioplasty and radial forearm flap phalloplasty in female-to-male transgender genital reconstruction: Is the "ideal" neophallus an achievable goal? Plastic and Reconstructive Surgery Global Open. 2016 Dec;**4**(12):e1131. DOI: 10.1097/gox.0000000000001131

[18] Santucci RA. Urethral complications after transgender phalloplasty: Strategies to treat them and minimize their occurrence. Clinical Anatomy. 2018;**31**(2):187-190

[19] Kim SK, Moon JB, Heo J, Kwon YS, Lee KC. A new method of urethroplasty for prevention of fistula in female-to male gender reassignment surgery. Annals of Plastic Surgery. 2010;**64**(6):759-764

[20] Levine LA, Elterman L. Urethroplasty following total phallic reconstruction. The Journal of Urology. 1998;**160**(2):378-382

[21] Jun MS, Santucci RA. Urethral stricture after phalloplasty. Translational Andrology and Urology. 2019;**8**(3):266

Chapter 8

Effects of Hypothalamic Blockers in the Treatment of Gender Dysphoria in Preadolescence: Medical and Psychological Implications of Taking Care

Massimo Di Grazia and Camilla Taverna

Abstract

Gender identity does not always develop in line with biological sex. Gender dysphoria at young age implies a strong incongruence between gender identity and the assigned sex; the rejection of one's sexual attributes and the desire to belong to the opposite sex; and a significant clinical suffering or impaired individual functioning in life spheres. The purpose of this chapter is a narrative review of the literature available on puberty suppression therapy through GnRH analogues. Biological puberty provides intense suffering to the adolescent with gender dysphoria who does not recognize himself in his own body. These drugs suppress the production of endogenous gametes and sex hormones. Although the effects of therapy are reversible, and biological development resumes spontaneously once the medication is stopped, the administration of GnRH analogues at a young age has fueled a scientific debate on the matter of the ethics of pharmacological intervention with minors. In conclusion, the studies considered show that GnRH analogues do not have long-term harmful effects on the body; prevent the negative psychosocial consequences associated with gender dysphoria in adolescence (suicidal ideation and attempts, self-medication, prostitution, self-harm); improve the psychological functioning of young transsexuals; and are diagnostic tools that allow adolescents to buy time to explore their gender identities.

Keywords: gender dysphoria, puberty suppression, GnRH analogues, preadolescence, AMAB, AFAB

1. Introduction

Gender identity was first defined by Stoller as "a complex system of beliefs that everyone has about himself, that is, his own sense of masculinity or femininity" [1]. According to the current binary system, which rigidly distinguishes male and female, the common expectation is that gender identity in children and adolescents develops in line with biological sex [2]. However, the developmental trajectories of gender identity are manifold. Only recently has a theorization of gender identity begun as a fluid dimension of the self, in which the boundaries between masculine and feminine are blurred, and of which diversified manifestations are possible [2]. In the case of young gender variants, interests and attitudes do not conform to the social stereotypes of masculinity and femininity [3]. If the gender variance is associated with clinically significant suffering, for which the young person shows a rejection of their sexual attributes and the desire to belong to the other gender, then it is gender dysphoria [4]. Gender dysphoria is a clinical condition and requires specialist intervention, which includes psychological care of the young person and the family, associated with targeted medical and pharmacological treatment [5]. Biological puberty generates severe suffering for adolescents with gender dysphoria who do not recognize themselves in their bodies and can interfere with psychological functioning and individual well-being. Drug therapies are currently available to alleviate the psychological distress associated with gender dysphoria. Suppression of biological puberty involves the administration of gonadotropin-releasing hormone (GnRH) analogues that disrupt the endogenous production of gametes and sex hormones, arresting the development of secondary sexual attributes [5–7]. However, the question of early pharmacological intervention with adolescents with gender dysphoria is still the subject of debate among professionals in the field, and further investigations are needed to better understand the benefits and risks associated with the therapy.

2. Puberty suppression

Hypothalamic blockers have been used in the treatment of children and adolescents with central precocious puberty since 1981. Empirical studies demonstrate the efficacy and long-term safety of similar drugs, such as gonadotropin-releasing hormone (GnRH) [8]. In 2009, the Endocrine Society published guidelines for the treatment of adolescents with gender dysphoria, recommending suppression of puberty with hypothalamic blocking drugs for patients who have reached Tanner stages 2–3 (Table 6 and Table 7 in the appendix) and who meet the eligibility criteria (further detailed below), assigning pediatricians to care for children with gender dysphoria [6]. The World Professional Association for Transgender Health also follows the Endocrine Society guidelines for the treatment of children and adolescents, and published the seventh edition of the Standards of Care [7]. Adolescents with gender dysphoria often consider the physical changes associated with puberty to be unsustainable [6, 9]. Girls experience breast appearance, followed by an increase in breast volume and fat mass. Breast growth is also associated with accelerated height development, with menarche usually occurring 2 years later. In boys, the first physical change is the growth of the testicles that reach a volume of at least 4 ml. Starting from a testicular volume of 10 ml, daily testosterone levels increase, resulting in virilization of the physical appearance. Physical changes in pubertal development are the consequence of the maturation of the hypothalamus-pituitary-gonadal axis and the development of secondary sexual characteristics [10]. According to clinical practice guidelines, transgender and gender non-conforming (TGNC) young people can undergo puberty suspension procedures, with the administration of the synthetic hormones GnRH analogues that have the effect of suppressing the endogenous production of sex hormones [6, 7, 11, 12]. The suppression of the functioning of the gonads can be effectively achieved with the inhibition of gonadotropic secretion with

GnRH analogues and antagonists [6]. While similar drugs achieve this effect after a short period of administration, the antagonists immediately block pituitary secretions. Since long-acting antagonists are not available for use in pharmacotherapy, long-acting agonist analogues are the best treatment option.

2.1 Eligibility criteria for treatment with gonadotropin-releasing hormone GnRH analogues

According to the indications provided in the Standards of Care, withdrawal therapy can only be started at the beginning of puberty, which coincides with Tanner stages 2–3 [7], and a detectable presence of steroid sex hormones in the blood [5]. The treatment eligibility criteria proposed in the Standards of Care are shown in **Table 1** [7].

2.2 Pharmacology of GnRH analogues

GnRH is a decapeptide produced by the GnRH-secreting neuronal system, located in the preoptic area of the anterior hypothalamus and the mid-basal hypothalamus [13]. The axons of GnRH secreting neurons send projections to different areas of the nervous system. Some of these terminate in a ganglion of vascular buttons in the median eminence of the primary portal vessel, which releases GnRH into gonadotropic cells. GnRH reaches the anterior pituitary via the portal system and activates specific receptors, stimulating the production of gonadotropins, such as luteinizing hormone (LH) and follicle-stimulating hormone (FSH). The gonadotropins thus synthesized regulate the activity of the gonads (reproductive organs), responsible for the production of gametes and female and male steroids. If GnRH is administered it results in rapid production of LH and less secretion of FSH. Since GnRH is a decapeptide, it is made up of a chain of 10 amino acids, joined together by a peptide bond. The amino acids of GnRH with crucial functions are found at positions 1, 2, 3, 6, and 10. A large number of analogues with agonistic or antagonistic properties have been synthesized, obtained by modifications of the amino acid chain. Triptorelin in GnRH analogue is mostly used to treat adolescents with gender dysphoria.

2.3 Pharmacodynamics

The single administration of GnRH agonists causes the secretion of LH and FSH in the pituitary cells, with the consequent regulation of the activity of the gonads

• The adolescent showed an intense and lasting pattern of gender non-compliance, or gender dysphoria (repressed or expressed);
• Gender dysphoria emerged or worsened at the onset of puberty;
• Any other coexisting psychological, social, medical problem (which could interfere with treatment) has been resolved, and the situation and functioning of the adolescent are sufficiently stable to be able to start therapy;
• The adolescent has provided informed consent, and especially when the patient has not reached the age to consent to medical procedures, the parents, or other caregivers or guardians, have consented to the treatment and/or are committed to offering support throughout the duration of the treatment process.

Table 1.
Eligibility criteria for treatment with GnRH analogues [7].

(stimulating or flare-up effect), [13]. Repeated administrations, on the other hand, result in the desensitization of gonadotropic cells and a reduction in the number of GnRH receptors on the membranes (down-regulation), with the effect of inhibiting the production of the hormones LH and FSH. The result is the blocking of the synthesis of androgens, estrogens, and male and female gametes. The mechanism of action of the antagonists is different since they act by blocking the pituitary receptors for endogenous GnRH and exogenous agonists, blocking access. Levels of LH and FSH decrease rapidly a few hours after administration. The drugs are effective in suppressing gonadotropic production, however, long-acting formulations have not yet been synthesized.

3. Criticism of pharmacological therapy

There are potential risks concerning the use of similar GnRH drugs, in relation to the effects that they can generate in the critical time interval for the development of the adolescent brain and bone mass. Although the therapy is safe in patients with central precocious puberty, these data are not generalizable to transsexual adolescents. For them, the treatment, in addition to starting later in development and continuing until the age of 15–16, is not followed by a process of inducing puberty of the biological sex, but of the opposite sex to that of birth [11]. These practices may also expose individuals to greater psychosocial difficulties as they remain physically prepubertal as peers reach puberty [5]. Therapy can thus contribute to more and more socially isolating transsexual adolescents, further increasing the risk of being victims of discrimination and bullying. Furthermore, adolescents could interpret the administration of hypothalamic blockers as a guarantee for future surgical sex reassignment, without engaging in other reflections on the matter [14]. They may risk feeling trapped in a certain life trajectory once puberty suppression therapy has begun, because family members and healthcare professionals, albeit in a benevolent way, may inadvertently reinforce a specific gender identity [12]. Furthermore, GnRH analogues are very expensive and not always reimbursed by health insurers [6, 9]. Progestins represent a less effective but more affordable alternative: they suppress gonadotropic secretion and exert a mild peripheral anti-androgen effect in boys; in girls, they suppress ovulation and progesterone production for long periods of time, with variable estrogen residues [15]. However, side effects such as disruption of adrenal functioning and bone growth are frequent at these doses of administration [6]. Therefore, when the patient can bear the costs of the therapy, the guidelines recommend proceeding with the administration of GnRH analogues, as they are safer and more effective [7].

4. Benefits of treatment with GnRH analogues

Empirical studies demonstrate the efficacy of GnRH analogue therapy in suppressing puberty in transgender adolescents. Schagen and colleagues found the efficacy of GnRH analogue therapy in suppressing puberty in trans adolescents: after 12 months of therapy, in 49 trans assigned female at birth (AFAB, mean age 13.6 years) adolescents, testicular development was halted with a reduction in volume, in 67 trans assigned male at birth (AMAB) adolescents, (mean age 14.2 years), menstruation was blocked and breast development regressed [16]. They share the belief that therapy is a way to allow patients to buy time in which they can mature cognitively and emotionally, in order to better manage gender variance [17]. In addition, the timeliness of the intervention is fundamental: hypothalamic blockers are less effective in reducing secondary sexual attributes when taken when puberty is already advanced (Tanner stage 4 or 5), [18]. If administered in prepuberty, drugs reduce the number of operations required in the future for gender reassignment, including breast removal in MtoF transsexual individuals, facial and voice feminization procedures in FtoM individuals [9, 19]. The cartilage of the nose, jaw, and larynx (Adam's apple) is also less developed after treatment [9, 20]. Those who are in favor of early treatment emphasize the suffering of patients who have been treated as adults, the advantage of buying time in the diagnostic phase, and having a physical appearance more conforming to that of the desired gender [11]. Also in Italy, a group of psychologists and endocrinologists expert in gender identity issues has begun to question the use of analogous GnRH drugs, coming to the conclusion that they do not cause any sex change, which temporarily suspends the formation of secondary sexual characteristics and have reversible effects [21]. Early therapy does not initiate the transition phase, but allows the adolescent to explore their gender identity, preventing, in the case of "desistant" young people in whom gender dysphoria would tend to regress naturally, the possibility of undergoing treatments more irreversible such as therapies with gender-affirming hormones (GAH) [9, 18, 19]. Adolescents have the opportunity to explore their gender identity in greater tranquility, without having to worry about the development of secondary sexual attributes [22]. Therapy with hypothalamic blockers can be considered a diagnostic tool since it allows a greater understanding of the degree and persistence of adolescent distress [23] and improves the accuracy of the diagnosis itself [20].

Another advantage of the use of GnRH analogues is the reversibility of the treatment: when the patient, after having explored the role consistent with gender identity, no longer wishes to undergo sex reassignment therapies, therapy with GnRH analogues can be interrupted and normal pubertal physiological development resumes [6, 19]. Furthermore, in adolescents who are already biologically mature but are undecided about cross-sex hormone therapy, hypothalamic blockers can inhibit those physiological functions that are perceived as unpleasant, such as menstruation in girls and erections in boys, in the intervening period, until the actual decision [11]. Regarding the efficacy of the drugs, the suppression of the activation of the hypothalamic–pituitary-gonadal axis has been demonstrated, with a reduction in testicular volume, in the levels of gonadotropins and prepubertal steroid sex hormones [23].

4.1 Psychological effects of the drug

Some international scientific societies, such as the World Professional Association for Transgender Health-WPATH; the European Society of Endocrinology-ESE; the European Society for Pediatric Endocrinology-ESPE; and the Lawson Wilkins Pediatric Endocrine Society-LWPES, recommend treatment with blockers that can improve children's quality of life and social relationships since gender-variant adolescents can experience severe distress that can lead to suicide [21]. Studies showing an association between the suspension of puberty and a reduction in depression and anxiety are encouraging in this regard [11, 12]. A better psychosocial adaptation seems to be related to early intervention, as the physical aspect more conforming to that of the experienced gender, allows one to be better accepted as a member of the other sex than those who start treatment in adulthood [20, 24]. Two longitudinal studies conducted by researchers from the medical centre of VU University in Amsterdam investigated the effectiveness of drug therapy with similar GnRH, in terms of psychological effects and drug tolerance. The first survey involved 70 transsexual adolescents [25]. The initiation of treatment was associated with reduced emotional and behavioral problems and an improvement in general functioning. However, the feelings of anger and anxiety remained stable even in a second measurement time before the start of cross-sex hormone therapy. The second research with 55 young transsexuals evaluated the long-term efficacy of the treatment protocol in subsequent times: before the start of therapy with GnRH analogues, at the time of induction of puberty with cross-sex hormones, 1 year after gender reassignment surgery [26]. By investigating psychological functioning and general well-being in areas such as social interactions and education or quality of life, the researchers showed that among young adults, gender dysphoria was attenuated, with improved psychological functioning following the beginning of gender-affirming medical interventions. Greater satisfaction with one's physical appearance was noted: the therapy had allowed an anatomical development that conformed to and not in contrast with one's gender identity. Furthermore, the psychological well-being level of the population was equal to or greater than that of the general population [26]. The results suggest that the origin of psychiatric symptoms may not be primarily psychiatric, but secondary to gender dysphoria, in particular, due to the development of secondary sexual attributes in the pubertal phase [26]. These results were replicated by a study conducted with young patients with gender dysphoria at Boston hospital [18]. Costa and colleagues [27] have evaluated the psychological functioning, measured with CGAS, in a sample of adolescents with gender dysphoria at different stages of care: after 6 months of psychological support; after 12 months of psychological support and six of treatment with similar GnRH; after 18 months of psychological support and 12 months of treatment with GnRH analogues using the Children's Global Assessment Scale (CGAS). The sample was divided into a group immediately eligible for treatment, and a group not immediately eligible for treatment. Young people immediately eligible for treatment had higher psychological functioning scores at the start of management and showed no significant improvement after 6 months of psychological support. Psychological functioning improved significantly after 12 months of treatment with GnRH analogues in young people immediately eligible for treatment, with results similar to those found in a sample of adolescents without psychological or psychiatric symptoms. On the other hand, in the group not immediately eligible for treatment, there was an improvement in functioning already after 6 months of psychological support. A 2011 study by the Dutch group evaluated psychological functioning by administering the Minnesota Multiphasic Inventory-2 (MMPI-2) and Minnesota Multiphasic Inventory-Adolescent (MMPI-A) in a group of adults and adolescents requiring reassignment of type. Compared to adolescents, a higher percentage of adults were in the clinically significant range of scores on the Paranoia scale (49.8% vs. 18. 1%, χ^2 (1) = 26.641, pb0.001) and the Psychasthenia scale (36.9% vs. 13.3%, χ^2 (1) = 16.662, pb0.001), [28].

When adolescents and adults were compared for the number of total MMPI scales for which they achieved scores in the range of clinical significance, most adults (62.8%) had clinical relevance scores for two or more scales. Instead, most adolescents (67.5%) had clinical relevance scores for none or only one of the subscales (χ^2 (2) = 24.198, pb0.001). The authors speculate that the better functioning observed in adolescents compared to adults may also be associated with the timing of the assessment since they had not yet developed secondary sexual characteristics.

4.2 Negative psychosocial outcomes of untreated gender dysphoria in adolescence

Brain development patterns during puberty increase the likelihood of adopting risky behaviors, a typical characteristic of adolescents [29]. However, the decision to undertake a reassignment process is not immediate and usually derives from a deep-rooted desire already present years before the young person turns to specialized centres. Furthermore, given the presence of this variable of impulsivity, adolescents with gender dysphoria could react to the omission of care by adopting risky behaviors, such as prostitution [30] and self-harming behaviors, even going so far as to attempt suicide [31].

4.2.1 Harm reduction model

The Harm Reduction Model is configured as an alternative to the moral model and the disease model, focusing on the consequences of deviant behavior [30]. When it is no longer possible to work preventively and the young transsexual has already adopted risky behaviors, he is encouraged to reduce them by the mental health professional who provides him with information on the pros and cons of each type of conduct, in order to protect his health [30, 32].

4.2.2 Autolesionism, suicides' ideations and attempts

For many professionals who treat developmental gender dysphoria, the decision to administer GnRH analogues is based on the fear of a possible increased risk of suicide in untreated adolescents. In the literature, there is a greater risk of suicidal ideation and attempts among young transsexuals [31, 33–35]. Studies investigating suicidal risk factors in transgender and gender non-conforming youth (TGNC) have identified gender dysphoria, parental physical and verbal abuse, and body image concerns as predictors [36]. Research conducted in Europe and America shows that young people with gender dysphoria are more likely to have other coexisting mental health problems, resulting in anxiety, depression, and suicidal tendencies [12]. GnRH analogue therapy has been shown to reduce psychological distress in transsexual adolescents [25, 26], so it could be hypothesized that the administration of hypothalamic blockers can actually prevent the adoption of suicidal behaviors in the adolescent with gender dysphoria. Spack and colleagues (2012) examined a sample of 97 adolescents with gender dysphoria from the Gender Management Service (GeMS) between January 1998 and February 2010 [18]. The data collected indicate that among young people: 44.3% had a history of psychiatric diagnoses; 37.1% took psychiatric drugs; 21.6% had a history of self-injurious behavior. Specifically, 20 patients reported self-mutilation episodes, and nine had attempted suicide at least once. The authors found an improvement in psychological functioning after medical intervention, suggesting that the patient's psychiatric symptoms may be secondary to gender dysphoria. Grossman and D'Augelli investigated the ideas and suicide attempts in a group of 55 adolescents with gender dysphoria [31]. The results obtained indicate an association between suicidal risk and two aspects related to self-esteem: body weight and the perception of one's physical appearance by others. Transsexual people strive to change their bodies in order to be perceived externally in a way that is congruent with their gender identity [37]. The use of hypothalamic blockers to nullify the inconsistency between perceived gender and the development of secondary sexual attributes reduces the stress associated with gender role transition and provides the opportunity to socially present oneself as a member of the opposite sex [38]. However, most adolescents with gender dysphoria do not have access to the care and resources to be able to achieve this state of self-congruence and satisfaction for their own bodies [31]. Therefore, age-appropriate medical treatment with GnRH analogues and hormones could prevent self-harming behaviors, ideas, and suicide attempts in young transsexuals. Indeed, when adequate treatment cannot be offered, some adolescents may react by making suicide attempts [30].

4.2.3 Automedication

Adolescents often prefer to buy hormones and blockers illegally rather than go to a specialized clinic, especially if the professional requires the fulfillment of many criteria to be able to administer the therapy [30]. If the doctor refuses to prescribe the therapy or to correct the dosage and way of taking it, young transsexuals will probably continue to obtain the drugs in unconventional ways. The risk of psychological, social, and behavioral complications is greater if the administration is not guided by a specialist [30]. The injection of potentially toxic, low-quality drugs without medical supervision could expose the adolescent to unsatisfactory physical outcomes and health-threatening medical conditions, such as HIV, AIDS, and hepatitis. Teens may also be given silicone injections, increasing the risk of infections or other complications (discolouration of surrounding tissues, inflammation and silicone-induced pulmonary embolism). Furthermore, involvement in illegal buying practices can have judicial consequences for young people, with repercussions in terms of social stigma and further involvement in the criminal justice system in adulthood [12, 39]. Those who come from geographic areas where gender adjustment treatments are not available often need to emigrate in order to receive appropriate medical treatment [39]. Often these are young illegal immigrants for whom prostitution remains the only option available to earn the money needed to pay for healthcare [40]. Baltieri and colleagues report two case reports of adolescents with gender dysphoria in Brazil who engaged in prostitution to obtain enough money to illegally buy cross-sex hormones, after being denied treatment because they were not reaching age, minimum sufficient [30]. Hormonal drugs were not given as there are no laws in Brazil regulating the medical treatment of young trans people.

4.2.4 Psychological issues

Denial of treatment has irreversible psychological effects on the psychosexual development of the adolescent since he will never be able to experience puberty in line with his own gender identity. Transsexual adolescents often suffer more from not being able to experience puberty of the desired sex than from the inability to experience puberty of the sex assigned at birth in case of treatment with similar GnRH [24]. Retrospective studies conducted with transsexual adults indicate that psychological problems, such as anxiety and depression, often emerge during puberty as a consequence of the distress associated with the development of secondary sexual attributes [24]. Psychopathologies secondary to gender dysphoria can, therefore, be prevented if we intervene in time [28]. Unfavorable outcomes of surgical gender reassignment in adults appear to be associated with late treatment rather than early intervention [41, 42]. Studies evaluating the psychological functioning of adults and transsexual adolescents from the same clinic also found improved functioning among adolescents who had been treated early with hormone therapy [28, 38, 43]. The poorer psychological functioning in adults may result in part from the constant and lasting distress they have experienced throughout their lives. In fact, the omission of treatment can result in long-term psychosocial outcomes such as stigmatization and social isolation [24].

5. Atypical development with GnRH analogues

Given the effects of drugs on the body during treatment, the guidelines recommend monitoring the adolescent with auxological clinical evaluations (weight, height, body mass index, blood pressure, and Tanner stage) every 3–6 months, and evaluation hormones (LH, FSH, estradiol, testosterone, prolactin, and 25-OH vitamin D) to be repeated every 6–12 months for the first year of therapy [5].

5.1 Short-term collateral effects

Hypothalamic blockers are generally well tolerated, with the exception of possible hot flashes [23], fatigue, migraine, mood changes, injection pain, and abscesses [5]. Some cases of arterial hypertension following the administration of Triptorelin were observed in three male transsexual adolescents in a sample of 138 subjects [5, 44]; and in two treated patients, with complications in one out of two patients related to increased intracranial pressure, which resulted in a temporary interruption of treatment [45]. The increase in intracranial pressure is a very rare side effect, usually associated only with the analogue GnRH drug Leuprolide [46]. The consequences that the use of similar GnRH drugs can have on blood pressure require further investigation [11].

5.2 Long-term collateral effects

5.2.1 Fertility

From the available literature, it is noted that treatment with analogous GnRH has no negative effects on the fertility of younger patients who are treated before the age of 7 [47], indeed it seems to have a protective effect in patients with central precocious puberty [48]. In young male (biological sex) adolescents with gender dysphoria undergoing GnRH analogue therapy, sperm production and development of the reproductive system is insufficient for sperm cryopreservation [6]. However, sperm production can be induced by a spontaneous recovery in gonadotropin production after cessation of GnRH analogues, or by gonadotropin-stimulating treatment (associated with physical manifestations of testosterone production), [6].

5.2.2 Nervous system effects

The physiological reorganization of the central nervous system occurs during puberty, in particular the executive functions located in the prefrontal cortex develop [49]. What emerges from the studies conducted so far is that there are no undesirable effects on brain development for adolescents undergoing therapy with GnRH analogues and GAF: the brain functioning of young patients seems to replicate that of the general population [24]. No negative effects on executive function emerged in research [50]. However, further long-term investigations are needed to arrive at more conclusive data [11].

5.2.3 Effects on bones development

During puberty, bone mass increases, reaching its maximum density around 20–30 years of age [11]. Suspension of puberty in adolescence is associated with reduced bone mineral density (BMD) in adult men [6]. Some studies do not detect changes in BMD values during the period of administration of GnRH analogues [6]. Other data report stable values of bone mineral density during therapy, but with a decrease in zeta scores, and a resumption of bone mass accumulation at the start of cross-sex hormone therapy [23]. When BMD was assessed in the same adult sample, a delay in reaching peak bone mass was detected, since the loss of zeta scores was still partially present at the age of 22. William Malone, an American endocrinologist interested in puberty blockers, affirms that the drugs seem to halt the rapid increase in bone density, the expected rise that takes place typically in adolescence is delayed [51]. Van Coverden and colleagues observed an increase in bone mass in the long-term treatment of adolescents with gender dysphoria: during the administration of gender-affirming hormones (GAF) there is a recovery in bone mass accumulation following normal physiological development [52]. Therapy with GnRH analogues appears to initially reduce BMD, with a future normalization after the induction of puberty with cross-sex hormones. Dutch studies report a reduction of BMD during puberty suppression, with a subsequent increase at the start of GAH therapy and achieving a final BMD no different than that observed before initiating analogue [44, 53].

5.2.4 Metabolical effects

The first data on early hormone therapy in adolescents with gender dysphoria revealed an increase in fat mass and a decrease in lean mass, only during the first year of treatment with Triptorelin, followed by a restoration of normal values with the administration of GAF [23]. Effects on lipid and carbohydrate metabolism were absent in the sample examined. Evidence shows an increase in body mass index (BMI) [54], an increase in fat mass, and a reduction in lean mass [16] in trans adolescents taking GnRH analogues.

5.2.5 Effects on growth

Suppression of puberty can impair growth in trans adolescents AFAB and AMAB [6, 55]. Schagen and colleagues found a reduction in the rate of growth rate in the sample of trans adolescents analyzed [16]. This can be an advantage for trans AMAB adolescents, who are more likely to reach a height similar to the average female population. Growth reduction can also have side effects on bone development and metabolism [56]. Subsequent therapy with cross-sex hormones allows for manipulation of growth and the achievement of an almost normal height [23]. Since the expected height for trans AMAB adolescents is greater than the female average, it is possible to increase the dose of estrogen administered during therapy with GAF, to reduce the final height. On the contrary, for trans AFAB adolescents, treatment with GnRH analogues must be longer, before being able to administer androgens at the age of 16 [55]. To achieve maximum height, a slow introduction of androgens mimics an acceleration of growth typical of puberty, or one can proceed with the administration of oxandrolone, a growth-stimulating anabolic steroid [6].

5.2.6 *Effects on venous circulation*

Despite the lack of clear results, venous thromboembolism can be a complication of drugs, so early screening for thrombophilia is appropriate for those with a personal or family history of venous thromboembolism [6].

6. Ethical aspects

The biomedical ethics model, theorized by Beauchamp and Childress, is the main point of reference for the management of ethical problems in the clinical setting [57]. According to the authors, there are four prerequisites that healthcare and health professionals must abide by in clinical practice, which are autonomy, non-maleficence, beneficence, and justice.

6.1 Autonomy

Hormonal treatment in puberty is justified as it aims to satisfy the desire of adolescents who want to align biological sex with their gender identity. Respect for the autonomy of the young person and the decision to undergo therapy should be emphasized, as the same results are not achievable if the drugs are administered in adulthood, except with invasive operations [20]. Furthermore, to fully respect the autonomy of the child, it is essential to educate him to know the different treatment options for gender dysphoria, in order to allow an informed decision, regardless of geographic location or socioeconomic status. The exercise of autonomy in the decision-making process is based on the recognition of children's rights and the informed consent expressed by the adolescent and the family [58].

6.2 Non-maleficence

The principle of non-maleficence imposes the obligation not to inflict harm on the patient. Hypothalamic blockers are classified as a reversible treatment since they appear to be free of long-term side effects. The doctor who respects the principle of non-maleficence adopts a more holistic approach and considers not only the possible damage to the body but also any negative consequences on the emotional, social, and spiritual values. For many adolescents, the ability to reduce the distress associated with developing secondary sexual attributes is far more important than drug-induced fertility deprivation. In general, the arguments against the use of blockers are based on the concern that gender dysphoria in childhood may go into remission in adolescence [59, 60]; on the impossibility of making a certain diagnosis of gender dysphoria in developmental age given the variability of gender identity in childhood and adolescence [17, 33]; and on the lack of knowledge of the long-term effects on the organism and psychological functioning [60, 61]. Furthermore, therapy can inhibit the spontaneous formation of a compliant gender identity, which sometimes develops through the "gender crisis" [62], and reduce libido, negatively affecting the adolescent's sexual experiences and limiting exploration of one's sexual orientation [17, 33]. Finally, for trans adolescents AMAB, the arrest of the development of the penis and testicles reduces the amount of skin tissue needed to perform a better vaginoplasty [63]. According to Giordano, the ethics of puberty suppression therapy depend not only on the balance of risks and benefits of the treatment but also on the evaluation of the consequences of the omission of treatment [39]. Health professionals must consider the long-term implications on the body (invasiveness of surgery), and the psychological and social/relational risks (self-loathing, social integration, and suicide risk).

6.3 Beneficence

Given the variability in the persistence of gender dysphoria from childhood to adulthood, it is not easy to establish how the specialist can operate in such a way as to respect the principle of beneficence The health professional makes some choices also influenced by personal belief systems and theoretical orientation that can influence the future of the adolescent, in both cases of treatment with similar GnRH and abstention from therapy [64]. The Standards of Care authorizes specialists to adapt the guidelines according to the needs and wishes of the individual patient [7]. The choice of prescribing blockers is ethical when the doctor believes that the patient will benefit from the treatment. If, after conducting the appropriate assessments, the physician concludes that refusal of treatment is the riskiest option because gender dysphoria is likely to persist into adolescence and adulthood, then early treatment is found to be in the best interests of the patient. Child [19]. The doctor's responsibility is to help the child or adolescent consider the possible consequences of each choice.

6.4 Justice

According to the principle of justice of Beauchamp and Childress, health services must be equally distributed among the population. Gender-dysphoric young people seeking assistance face a variety of barriers due to socioeconomic status and geographic location. There are disparities in access to care between gender-variant adolescents and cisgender peers, due to the stigma that prevents them from seeking and obtaining adequate treatments [12]. The social and structural stigma experienced by gender non-conforming young people reduces accessibility to care from a structural, interpersonal, and individual point of view [65]. The structural stigma implies a reduction in available resources and health coverage; the medicalization of atypical expressions of gender identity; electronic registers with only two options for gender identification; the lack of knowledge and research on the health of trans people [65]. Stigma in social relationships at school and in the family also represents a barrier to access to specialized medical services for atypical gender identity [66]. Young people, inserted in a stigmatizing social context, are increasingly reluctant to reveal their atypical gender identity. The tendency to hide associated with the fear of being judged as different reduces the likelihood for young gender-variant people to seek and receive assistance [67]. Furthermore, the services are not equally distributed throughout the territory, so there are few clinics with specialized professionals who are used to treat problems related to gender identity, generating inequalities in access to care due to geographic location. The shortage of adequately trained and competent personnel can lead to inappropriate or even harmful medical care for patients [68]. Gender-variant young people often have difficulty accessing other forms of assistance [69].

7. Conclusion

The experience of biological puberty is an undesirable condition for adolescents with gender dysphoria who find themselves living in a body they do not recognize as their own. Actionable interventions for gender dysphoria are classified in the Standards of Care as fully reversible, partially reversible, and irreversible interventions [7]. Suppression of puberty is a reversible treatment that involves the administration of similar drugs of gonadotropin-releasing hormone (GnRH). The analogue agonist most frequently used with adolescents with gender dysphoria is Triptorelin, administered by the intramuscular or subcutaneous route. This intervenes to arrest the development of secondary sexual attributes and associated physiological functions in adolescents with gender dysphoria. After the suppression of puberty, if gender dysphoria persists, the induction of puberty of gender identification can be carried out by administering GAF [11]. Regarding drug safety, GnRH analogues appear to be well tolerated in the short term, with the exception of hot flashes [23], fatigue, migraine, mood swings, pain from injection, and abscesses [5]. Even in the long term, there do not seem to be any significant side effects on the body, but the knowledge is still uncertain [11]. The issue of fertility is particularly delicate, since, if the gender adjustment process is continued, it remains irremediably compromised for adolescents who have not resorted to the preservation of sexual gametes. This aspect represents an element to be evaluated when defining the decision-making capacity of the minor who chooses to undergo medical treatment for gender dysphoria [24]. When the young person has not yet reached the age of majority, the request for the gender adjustment process should be accompanied by parental approval. However, there is no agreement on the minimum age for adolescents to express consent. Furthermore, it seems useless to establish an age threshold: the International Covenant on the Rights of the Child focuses on the capacity for judgment, whereby the adolescent can express consent when he has reached sufficient emotional and cognitive maturity to understand the implications of therapy, including possible side effects and risks that may occur [12]. Since puberty suppression therapy is partly experimental, consent cannot be fully informed, because the professionals themselves are not aware of all the long-term outcomes of drugs on the body [19]. The candidate can undertake treatment if he meets the eligibility criteria for treatment, whereby the professional assesses whether the adolescent is able to understand and provide consent; and was informed of the expected outcomes, possible disadvantages, potential loss of fertility, and opportunities for preserving fertility [5].

Parents have the right to make decisions for their children only when they do not hinder the "best interests" of young people [12]. The choice of the clinician should not be based only on parental opinion, because parents do not always know what their children's wishes are, and there is a risk of limiting the child's right to autonomy [17]. Gender dysphoria implies a strong inconsistency between assigned sex and experienced gender, with a rejection of one's sexual attributes leading to clinically significant suffering and impaired individual functioning in daily life [4]. This condition is also associated with problems of a psychological and psychiatric nature, such as depression and anxiety [70]; suicide ideas and attempts [18, 31, 35]; an intense dissatisfaction with one's body image [71, 72].

The negative psychosocial consequences of untreated gender dysphoria in adolescence are now well known. First of all, the young person can experience the omission of treatment as psychological torture and interpret it as a denial of the possibility of experiencing puberty of the kind of identification. Faced with this suffering, the adolescent who reacts with impulsiveness can adopt behaviors that are risky to health [30]. The anguish can be so intense that it leads to suicidal ideas and attempts. Suicidal behaviors are more frequent in the transgender population than in the rest of the population [31, 33–35]. Unfavorable outcomes of surgical gender reassignment in adults appear to be associated with late treatment rather than early intervention [41]. Poorer psychological functioning in adults could be due to the distress experienced due to a prolonged inconsistency between gender identity and physical appearance that exposes to stigmatization and social isolation [24]. On the other hand, timely treatment with similar GnRH not only allows to prevent negative outcomes but also bring benefits to the young person. The same effects cannot be obtained if therapy is started later in puberty, as blockers are less effective in reducing secondary sexual attributes when they are already formed [18, 20], for which it will be necessary to expose themselves to invasive surgical removal operations in the future. Suppression of puberty can be considered a diagnostic tool, as it saves time for both the adolescent, who can explore their gender identity without worrying about the development of secondary sexual attributes [22], and to the clinician, who can better understand the nature and intensity of adolescent distress [23] to arrive at a more precise diagnosis [20]. Many studies have found an improvement in functioning and psychological well-being after treatment with GnRH analogues [25–38]. When, on the other hand, therapy is denied, and the adolescent resorts to self-medication, he is no longer followed by professionals in the sector, with the foreseeable physical and psychological repercussions that follow (wrong methods and dosages of administration, possible infections due to injections that do not comply with appropriate hygiene standards), [12, 39]. Involvement in prostitution exposes adolescents to situations that are risky for their life and sexual health since they could be victims of abuse or contract infections and diseases if they do not use the appropriate precautions [71]. The advantages that can be brought by GnRH analogue therapy cannot be underestimated, which are arresting in the development of secondary sexual attributes and greater satisfaction with body image; preventing a series of risky behaviors for health, in particular suicidal ideations and attempts. The right of the adolescent emerges to a future in which life opportunities are maximized, whereby the possibility of living the puberty experience of gender identification is offered, preventing the need to undergo invasive gender affirmation surgeries in future [73–75]. The importance of respecting the right of the child to exercise personal autonomy in the decision-making process is noted, so his/her opinion must be considered by the professional when making a therapeutic choice [17, 76, 77]. Whether parents not only deny consent but adopt abusive attitudes towards the gender-variant child, then the possibility of intervention to protect the minor is evaluated [78]. Since the prevalence of gender in adolescence is progressively increasing in the population [24], this issue cannot be underestimated, and it is important to convey the right therapeutic tools for young people afferent to health services [79]. It is clear that denial of therapy is not a neutral option, and the health professional cannot omit the intervention, thus thinking of not harming the patient. This type of action can harm young people in two ways: it does not respect the principle of non-maleficence as they can adopt risk behaviors that compromise their health; does not respect the principle of beneficence as it does not bring benefit. The studies cited highlight the importance of evaluating for each case which therapeutic option is that can improve the well-being and quality of life of the minor, without focusing on rigid and a priori beliefs, but keeping the multiple possibilities of treatment open.

Author details

Massimo Di Grazia[1] and Camilla Taverna[2]*

1 Hospital Infermi, AUSL Romagna, Rimini, Italy

2 University of Padova, Padova, Italy

*Address all correspondence to: camillataverna5@gmail.com

References

[1] Stoller R. Sex and Gender. On the development of masculinity and femininity. New York: Science House; 1968.

[2] Massara D, Baietto C, Di Grazia M, Finzi S, Manzon M, Caldarera A. La disforia di genere nell'infanzia. In: Graglia M, editor. Rivista di Sessuologia. Roma: Scioni Editore; 2016. pp. 40(2): 108-40(2):122

[3] Steensma TD. From Gender Variance to Gender Dysphoria: Psychosexual development of gender atypical children and adolescents [PhD-thesis]. Amsterdam: Vrije Universiteit Amsterdam; 2013

[4] American Psychiatric Association. Diagnostic and Statistical Manual of Mental Disorders. 5th ed. Washington: American Psychiatric Press; 2013

[5] Hembree WC, Cohen-Kettenis PT, Gooren L, Hannema SE, Meyer WJ, Murad MH, et al. Endocrine treatment of gender-dysphoric/gender-incongruent persons: An endocrine society clinical practice guideline. The Journal of Clinical Endocrinology and Metabolism. 2017;**102**(11):3869-3903

[6] Hembree WC, Cohen-Kettenis P, Delemarre-van de Waal HA, Gooren LJ, Meyer WJ 3rd, Spack NP, et al. Endocrine Society. Endocrine Treatment of Transsexual Persons: An Endocrine Society Clinical Practice Guideline. The Journal of Clinical Endocrinology and Metabolism. 2009;**94**(9):3132-3154

[7] WPATH. Standards of care for the health of transexual, transgender and gender nonconforming people. Version 7. International Journal of Transgenderism. 2011;**13**:165-232

[8] Carel JC, Eugster EA, Rogol A, Ghizzoni L, Palmert MR, ESPE-LWPES GnRH Analogs Consensus Conference Group, et al. Consensus statement on the use of gonadotropin-releasing hormone analogs in children. Pediatrics. 2009;**123**(4):752-762. DOI: 10.1542/peds.2008-1783

[9] Fisher AD, Ristori J, Bandini E, Giordano S, Mosconi M, Jannini EA, et al. Medical treatment in gender dysphoric adolescents endorsed by SIAMS-SIE-SIEDP-ONIG. Journal of Endocrinological Investigation. 2014;**37**(7):675-687. DOI: 10.1007/s40618-014-0077-6

[10] Bakker J. Sex differentiation: Organizing effects of sex hormones. In: Kreukels BPC, Steensma TD, de Vries ALC, editors. Focus on Sexuality Research. Gender Dysphoria and Disorders of Sex Development: Progress in Care and Knowledge. New York: Springer; 2014. p. 3-24. DOI: 10.1007/978-1-4614-7441-8_1

[11] Cohen-Kettenis PT, Klink D. Adolescents with gender dysphoria. Best Practice & Research Clinical Endocrinology & Metabolism. 2015;**29**(3): 485-495. DOI: 10.1016/j.beem.2015.01.004

[12] Kimberly LL, Folkers KM, Friesen P, Sultan D, Quinn GP, Bateman-House A, et al. Ethical issues in gender-affirming care for youth. Pediatrics. 2018;**142**(6):e20181537. DOI: 10.1542/peds.2018-1537

[13] Scarselli, G., Comparetto, C., & Coccia, M. E. (2006). Analoghi del GnRH: agonisti e antagonisti. In Di Renzo, G. (Eds.), Ginecologia e ostetricia, 1729-1744. Roma: Verducci

[14] Wren B. Early physical intervention for young people with atypical gender identity

development. Clinical Child Psychology and Psychiatry. 2000;5(2):220-231. DOI: 10.1177/1359104500005002007

[15] Meriggiola MC, Gava G. Endocrine care of transpeople part I. A review of cross-sex hormonal treatments, outcomes and adverse effects in transmen. Clinical Endocrinology. 2015;**83**(5):597-606. DOI: 10.1111/cen.12753

[16] Schagen SE, Cohen-Kettenis PT, Delemarre-van de Waal HA, Hannema SE. Efficacy and safety of gonadotropin-releasing hormone agonist treatment to suppress puberty in gender dysphoric adolescents. The Journal of Sexual Medicine. 2016;**13**(7):1125-1132. DOI: 10.1016/j.jsxm.2016.05.004

[17] Stein E. Commentary on the treatment of gender variant and gender dysphoric children and adolescents: Common themes and ethical reflections. Journal of Homosexuality. 2012;**59**(3):480-500. DOI: 10.1080/00918369.2012.653316

[18] Spack NP, Edwards-Leeper L, Feldman HA, Leibowitz S, Mandel F, Diamond DA, et al. Children and adolescents with gender identity disorder referred to a pediatric medical center. Pediatrics. 2012;**129**(3):418-425. DOI: 10.1542/peds.2011-0907

[19] Giordano S. Medical treatment for children with gender dysphoria. In: BPC K, Steensma TD, ALC d V, editors. Focus on Sexuality Research. Gender Dysphoria and Disorders of Sex Development: Progress in Care and Knowledge. New York: Springer; 2014. pp. 205-230. ISBN: 9781461474401

[20] Cohen-Kettenis PT, Pfafflin F. Transgenderism and Intersexuality in Childhood and Adolescence. Making Choices. London: SAGE Publications, Inc.; 2003

[21] Valerio P, Scandurra C, Amodeo A. Appunti sul Genere. In: Riflessioni sulle linee-guida di intervento psicologico e dintorni. Etica e buone prassi nella professione di psicologo. Napoli: Edizione Ordine Psicologi della Campania; 2015

[22] Zucker KJ, Bradley SJ, Owen-Anderson A, Kibblewhite SJ, Wood H, Singh D, et al. Demographics, behavior problems, and psychosexual characteristics of adolescents with gender identity disorder or transvestic fetishism. Journal of Sex & Marital Therapy. 2012;**38**(2):151-189. DOI: 10.1080/0092623X.2011.611219

[23] Delemarre-van de Waal HA, Cohen Kettenis PT. Clinical management of gender identity disorders in adolescents: a protocol on psychological and paediatric endocrinology aspects. European Journal of Endocrinology. 2006;**155**:131-137. DOI: 10.1530/eje.1.02231

[24] Kreukels BP, Cohen-Kettenis PT. Puberty suppression in gender identity disorder: The Amsterdam experience. Nature Reviews. Endocrinology. 2011;**7**(8):466-472. DOI: 10.1038/nrendo.2011.78

[25] de Vries ALC, Steensma TD, Doreleijers TA, Cohen-Kettenis PT. Puberty suppression in adolescents with gender identity disorder: A prospective follow-up study. The Journal of Sexual Medicine. 2011;**8**(8):2276-2283

[26] de Vries AL, McGuire JK, Steensma TD, Wagenaar EC, Doreleijers TA, Cohen-Kettenis PT. Young adult psychological outcome after puberty suppression and gender reassignment. Pediatrics. 2014;**134**(4):696-704. DOI: 10.1542/peds.2013-2958

[27] Costa R, Dunsford M, Skagerberg E, Holt V, Carmichael P, Colizzi M. Psychological support, puberty

suppression, and psychosocial functioning in adolescents with gender dysphoria. The Journal of Sexual Medicine. 2015;**12**(11):2206-2214. DOI: 10.1111/jsm.13034

[28] de Vries AL, Kreukels BP, Steensma TD, Doreleijers TA, Cohen-Kettenis PT. Comparing adult and adolescent transsexuals: an MMPI-2 and MMPI-A study. Psychiatry Research. 2011;**186**(2-3):414-418. DOI: 10.1016/j.psychres.2010.07.033

[29] Steinberg L. A behavioral scientist looks at the science of adolescent brain development. Brain and Cognition. 2010;**72**(1):160-164. DOI: 10.1016/j.bandc.2009.11.003

[30] Baltieri DA, Prado Cortez FC, de Andrade AG. Ethical conflicts over the management of transsexual adolescents--report of two cases. The Journal of Sexual Medicine. 2009;**6**(11):3214-3220. DOI: 10.1111/j.1743-6109.2009.01409.x

[31] Grossman AH, D'Augelli AR. Transgender youth and life-threatening behaviors. Suicide & Life-Threatening Behavior. 2007;**37**(5):527-537. DOI: 10.1521/suli.2007.37.5.527

[32] Sanchez NF, Sanchez JP, Danoff A. Health care utilization, barriers to care, and hormone usage among male-to-female transgender persons in New York City. American Journal of Public Health. 2009;**99**(4):713-719. DOI: 10.2105/AJPH.2007.132035

[33] Korte A, Lehmkuhl U, Goecker D, Beier KM, Krude H, Grüters-Kieslich A. Gender identity disorders in childhood and adolescence: Currently debated concepts and treatment strategies. Deutsches Ärzteblatt International. 2008;**105**(48):834-841. DOI: 10.3238/arztebl.2008.0834

[34] Skagerberg E, Parkinson R, Carmichael P. Self-harming thoughts and behaviors in a group of children and adolescents with gender dysphoria. International Journal of Transgenderism. 2013;**14**(2):86-92

[35] Holt V, Skagerberg E, Dunsford M. Young people with features of gender dysphoria: Demographics and associated difficulties. Clinical Child Psychology and Psychiatry. 2016;**21**(1):108-118. DOI: 10.1177/1359104514558431

[36] Simons L, Schrager SM, Clark LF, Belzer M, Olson J. Parental support and mental health among transgender adolescents. Journal of Adolescent Health. 2013;**53**(6):791-793. DOI: 10.1016/j.jadohealth.2013.07.019

[37] Green R. The behaviorally feminine male child: Pretranssexual? pretransvestic? pre-homosexual? reheterosexual? [thesis]. Washington: Washington State University (WSU); 1974

[38] Smith YL, Van Goozen SH, Kuiper AJ, Cohen-Kettenis PT. Sex reassignment: outcomes and predictors of treatment for adolescent and adult transsexuals. Psychological Medicine. 2005;**35**(1):89-99. DOI: 10.1017/s0033291704002776

[39] Giordano S. Ethics of management of gender atypical organisation in children and adolescents. In: Boylan M, editor. International Public Health Policy and Ethics. International Library of Ethics, Law, and the New Medicine. Vol. 42. New York: Springer; 2008. pp. 249-272

[40] Fernanda de Albuquerque F, Janelli M. Princesa. Roma: Sensibili alle Foglie; 1994

[41] Gijs L, Brewaeys A. Surgical treatment of gender dysphoria in adults and adolescents: Recent developments, effectiveness, and challenges. Annual Review of Sex Research. 2007;**18**:178-184. DOI: 10.1080/10532528.2007.10559851

[42] Pfäfflin F, Junge A. Sex Reassignment: Thirty Years of International Follow-Up Studies After Sex Reassignment Surgery: A Comprehensive Review, 1961-1991. Düsseldorf, Germany: Symposion; 2003. p. 2003

[43] Kuiper B, Cohen-Kettenis P. Sex reassignment surgery: a study of 141 Dutch transsexuals. Archives of Sexual Behavior. 1988;**17**(5):439-457. DOI: 10.1007/BF01542484

[44] Klink D, Caris M, Heijboer A, van Trotsenburg M, Rotteveel J. Bone mass in young adulthood following gonadotropin-releasing hormone analog treatment and cross-sex hormone treatment in adolescents with gender dysphoria. The Journal of Clinical Endocrinology and Metabolism. 2015;**100**(2):E270-E275. DOI: 10.1210/jc.2014-2439

[45] Jong A, Bökenkamp A, Klink D. Arterial hypertension as a complication of prolonged therapy with GnRH-analogues in adolescent girls. Klinische Pädiatrie. 2011;**223**(S 01). DOI: 10.1055/s-0031-1273887

[46] Arber N, Shirin H, Fadila R, Melamed E, Pinkhas J, Sidi Y. Pseudotumor cerebri associated with leuprorelin acetate. Lancet (London, England). 1990;**335**(8690):668. DOI: 10.1016/0140-6736(90)90460-m

[47] Heger S, Müller M, Ranke M, Schwarz HP, Waldhauser F, Partsch CJ, et al. Long-term GnRH agonist treatment for female central precocious puberty does not impair reproductive function. Molecular and Cellular Endocrinology. 2006;**254-255**:217-220. DOI: 10.1016/j.mce.2006.04.012

[48] Lazar L, Meyerovitch J, de Vries L, Phillip M, Lebenthal Y. Treated and untreated women with idiopathic precocious puberty: Long-term follow-up and reproductive outcome between the third and fifth decades. Clinical Endocrinology. 2014;**80**(4):570-576. DOI: 10.1111/cen.12319

[49] Huttenlocher PR. Synaptic density in human frontal cortex - developmental changes and effects of aging. Brain Research. 1979;**163**(2):195-205. DOI: 10.1016/0006-8993(79)90349-4

[50] Staphorsius AS, Kreukels BP, Cohen-Kettenis PT, Veltman DJ, Burke SM, Schagen SE, et al. Puberty suppression and executive functioning: An fMRI-study in adolescents with gender dysphoria. Psychoneuroendocrinology. 2015;**56**:190-199. DOI: 10.1016/j.psyneuen.2015.03.007

[51] Cohen D, Barnes H. Gender dysphoria in children: Puberty blockers study draws further criticism. Brithish Medical Journal. 2019;**366**:l5647. DOI: 10.1136/bmj.l5647

[52] van Coeverden SC, Netelenbos JC, de Ridder CM, Roos JC, Popp-Snijders C, Delemarre-van de Waal HA. Bone metabolism markers and bone mass in healthy pubertal boys and girls. Clinical Endocrinology. 2002;**57**(1):107-116. DOI: 10.1046/j.1365-2265.2002.01573.x

[53] Vlot MC, Klink DT, den Heijer M, Blankenstein MA, Rotteveel J, Heijboer AC. Effect of pubertal suppression and cross-sex hormone therapy on bone turnover markers and bone mineral apparent density (BMAD) in transgender adolescents. Bone. 2017;**95**: 11-19. DOI: 10.1016/j.bone.2016.11.008

[54] Wouters F, Schagen SE, Cohen-Kettenis PT, Delemarre-van de Waal HA. Long-term delay of puberty by treatment with GnRH analogues and the effect on bone mineral density in transsexual adolescents. Hormone Research. 2007;**68**(1):67

[55] Delemarre-Van de Waal HA. Early medical intervention in adolescents with gender dysphoria. In: BPC K, Steensma TD, ALC d V, editors. Focus on Sexuality Research. Gender Dysphoria and Disorders of Sex Development: Progress in Care and Knowledge. Vol. 2014. New York, NY: Springer; 2014. pp. 293-204

[56] Haraldsen IR, Haug E, Falch J, Egeland T, Opjordsmoen S. Cross-sex pattern of bone mineral density in early onset gender identity disorder. Hormones and Behavior. 2007;**52**:334-343. DOI: 10.1016/j.yhbeh.2007.05.012

[57] Beauchamp TL, Childress JF. Principles of Biomedical Ethics. 7th ed. New York: Oxford University Press; 2013

[58] Di Ceglie D. Autonomia e processo decisionale nel lavoro con bambini e adolescenti con disforia di genere. In: Graglia M, editor. Prospettive sui generis, sguardi psicosociali sulle varianze di genere. Rivista di Sessuologia. Roma: Scioni Editore; 2020. pp. 220-231

[59] Abel BS. Hormone treatment of children and adolescents with gender dysphoria: An ethical analysis. The Hastings Center Report. 2014;**44**(Suppl 4):S23-S27. DOI: 10.1002/hast.366

[60] Cohen-Kettenis PT, Delemarre-van de Waal HA, Gooren LJ. The treatment of adolescent transsexuals: Changing insights. The Journal of Sexual Medicine. 2008;**5**(8):1892-1897. DOI: 10.1111/j.1743-6109.2008.00870.x

[61] Drummond KD, Bradley SJ, Peterson-Badali M, Zucker KJ. A follow-up study of girls with gender identity disorder. Developmental Psychology. 2008;**44**(1):34-45. DOI: 10.1037/0012-1649.44.1.34

[62] Giordano S. Gender atypical organisation in children and adolescents: Ethico-legal Issues and a proposal for new guidelines. The International Journal of Children's Rights. 2007;**15**:365-390. DOI: 10.1163/092755607X262793

[63] Milrod C. How young is too young: Ethical concerns in genital surgery of the transgender MTF adolescent. The Journal of Sexual Medicine. 2014;**11**:338-346. DOI: 10.1111/jsm.12387

[64] Drescher J, Byne W. Gender dysphoric/gender variant (GD/GV) children and adolescents: summarizing what we know and what we have yet to learn. Journal of Homosexuality. 2012;**59**(3):501-510. DOI: 10.1080/00918369.2012.653317

[65] White Hughto JM, Reisner SL, Pachankis JE. Transgender stigma and health: A critical review of stigma determinants, mechanisms, and interventions. Social Science & Medicine. 2015;**147**:222-231. DOI: 10.1016/j.socscimed.2015.11.010

[66] Winter S, Diamond M, Green J, Karasic D, Reed T, Whittle S, et al. Transgender people: Health at the margins of society. Lancet (London, England). 2016;**388**(10042):390-400. DOI: 10.1016/S0140-6736(16)00683-8

[67] Roberts TK, Fantz CR. Barriers to quality health care for the transgender population. Clinical Biochemistry. 2014;**47**(10-11):983-987. DOI: 10.1016/j.clinbiochem.2014.02.009

[68] Wylie K, Knudson G, Khan SI, Bonierbale M, Watanyusakul S, Baral S. Serving transgender people: Clinical care considerations and service delivery models in transgender health. Lancet. 2016;**388**(10042):401-411. DOI: 10.1016/S0140-6736(16)00682-6

[69] Safer JD, Coleman E, Feldman J, Garofalo R, Hembree W, Radix A, et al. Barriers to healthcare for transgender

individuals. Current Opinion in Endocrinology, Diabetes, and Obesity. 2016;**23**(2):168-171. DOI: 10.1097/MED.0000000000000227

[70] de Vries AL, Doreleijers TA, Steensma TD, Cohen-Kettenis PT. Psychiatric comorbidity in gender dysphoric adolescents. Journal of Child Psychology and Psychiatry. 2011;**52**(11):1195-1202. DOI: 10.1111/j.1469-7610.2011.02426.x

[71] Hepp U, Milos G. Gender identity disorder and eating disorders. International Journal of Eating Disorders. 2002;**32**(4):473-478. DOI: 10.1002/eat.10090

[72] Surgenor LJ, Fear JL. Eating disorder in a transgendered patient: A case report. International Journal of Eating Disorders. 1998;**24**(4):449-452. DOI: 10.1002/(sici)1098-108x(199812)24:4<449::aid-eat14>3.0.co;2-w

[73] Martinerie L, Condat A, Bargiacchi A, Bremont-Weill C, de Vries MC, Hannema SE. Management of endocrine disease: Approach to the management of children and adolescents with gender dysphoria. European Journal of Endocrinology. 2018;**179**(5):R219-R237. DOI: 10.1530/EJE-18-0227

[74] Ehrensaft D. From gender identity disorder to gender identity creativity: True gender self child therapy. Journal of Homosexuality. 2012;**59**(3):337-356. DOI: 10.1080/00918369.2012.653303

[75] Edwards-Leeper L, Spack NP. Psychological evaluation and medical treatment of transgender youth in an interdisciplinary "Gender Management Service" (GeMS) in a major pediatric center. Journal of Homosexuality. 2012;**59**(3):321-336. DOI: 10.1080/00918369.2012.653302

[76] de Vries AL, Cohen-Kettenis PT. Clinical management of gender dysphoria in children and adolescents: the Dutch approach. Journal of Homosexuality. 2012;**59**(3):301-320. DOI: 10.1080/00918369.2012.653300

[77] de Vries AL, Noens IL, Cohen-Kettenis PT, van Berckelaer-Onnes IA, Doreleijers TA. Autism spectrum disorders in gender dysphoric children and adolescents. Journal of Autism and Developmental Disorders. 2010;**40**(8):930-936. DOI: 10.1007/s10803-010-0935-9

[78] Holman CW, Goldberg JM. Social and medical transgender case advocacy. International Journal of Transgenderism. 2007;**9**(3-4):197-217. DOI: 10.1300/J485v09n03_09

[79] Di Grazia M, Sammartano F, Taverna C, Knowles A, Trombetta C, Barbone F. Epidemiologic considerations on gender incongruence in adults, adolescents and children and mental health issues: A review of the literature. Sexologies. 2021;**30**(1):61-75. DOI: 10.1016/J.SEXOL.2020.12.003